Short cases for the
MRCP

Short cases for the MRCP

Charles R K Hind
BSc (Hons) MD MRCP

Consultant Physician, General and
Respiratory Medicine, Royal Liverpool
Hospital and Regional Adult Cardiothoracic
Unit, Broadgreen Hospital;
Clinical Lecturer in Medicine,
University of Liverpool

CHURCHILL LIVINGSTONE
EDINBURGH LONDON MELBOURNE AND NEW YORK 1984

CHURCHILL LIVINGSTONE
Medical Division of Longman Group UK Limited

Distributed in the United States of America by Churchill
Livingstone Inc., 1560 Broadway, New York, N.Y. 10036, and
by associated companies, branches and representatives
throughout the world.

First published 1984
    Reprinted 1986
    Reprinted 1987
    Reprinted 1988
    Reprinted 1989

ISBN 0 443 02941 5

British Library Cataloguing in Publication Data
Hind, C.R.K.
    Short cases for MRCP
    1. Medicine — Problems, exercises, etc
    I. Title
    610'.76   R834.5

Library of Congress Cataloging in Publication Data
Hind, Charles R. K. (Charles Robert Keith)
    Short cases for MRCP.

    Bibliography: p.
    Includes index.
    1. Diagnosis — Case studies. 2. Physical diagnosis —
Case studies. I. Title. II. Title: Short cases for
M.R.C.P. [DNLM: 1. Diagnosis — Examination questions
2. Physical examination — Examination questions. WB
18 H662s]
RC71.3.H56   1984   616.07'54   83-25167

Produced by Longman Singapore Publishers Pte Ltd
Printed in Singapore

Preface

The part of the MRCP (UK) examination which is
feared most is the clinical section; in particular, the
short cases, where the candidate's ability to elicit and
interpret physical signs is closely scrutinised by the
examiners. It is in this part of the examination that the
highest percentage of failures occurs. Some candidates
fail because they lack the necessary clinical competence
and knowledge. Many more fail because of inadequate
preparation, lack of technique and poor presentation.
Continued practice is the only way to correct these
faults, and no book can hope to replace this. A book
can, however, hasten this process and that is the aim of
this small volume. Within the 11 chapters are suggested
techniques for examining each system and region of the
body encountered as short cases. Throughout, the
emphasis is on those mistakes most often made by the
candidate, and the causes, other features and frequency
of presentation of each abnormal sign. In addition,
detailed descriptions are given of typical short cases
used in the MRCP examination. Many of these
disorders are rare in clinical practice, but often
encountered as short cases. Candidates should be
familiar with these, so they can make a 'spot diagnosis'.
The size of the book is such that it can be carried in the
pocket of a white coat and so be readily available at the
bedside for reference. Spaces are available in the text for
the reader to add his or her own particular reminders.

In such a small book the information contained
cannot be comprehensive, and assumes much basic
knowledge. If unfamiliar with any of the clinical
features referred to, candidates should consult one of
the standard textbooks or colour atlases listed in the
bibliography section. It is from these that much of the
detailed information included in this book is derived.

The idea of writing this book arose from my
experience in teaching MRCP candidates at the
Hammersmith Hospital. The comments on the relative
frequency of each sign or disorder as a short case are
based on later feedback from these candidates. If anyone
has any suggestions for improvements, I would happily
listen to them.

I would like to thank Dr Fiona Fraser for her practical guidance; the staff of Churchill Livingstone for their support; and Ms Denise Brinkman for her usual excellent Secretarial assistance.

London, 1984   C.R.K.H.

Contents

1. General approach

INTRODUCTION *'You are not expected to be encyclopaedic, but polished in technique, professional in your approach, safe in practice and honest in ignorance.'*

(J Constable 1975 *Update* 1 : 635)

The short cases section of the MRCP (UK) examination consists of a 30 minute period in which you are asked to examine six or more patients in front of two examiners. Such examination is either 'blind' (e.g. 'Listen to this patient's heart'), or based on some clinical information (e.g. 'Examine this patient with hypertension'). After examining the patient, you are asked to present your findings, suggest a suitable diagnosis or list of differential diagnoses, and perhaps describe some other features of the particular sign or disorder. The aim of this part of the examination is threefold:

1. To assess your skill in examining a patient. You should be quick, gentle and thorough. During the run-up to the examination you should perfect techniques for examining every system and region of the body, in a manner which appears as second nature to you. Only practice makes perfect, preferably in front of a consultant or registrar under 'examination conditions'.

2. To test your judgement. That is, your ability to adapt these techniques to determine the cause of a particular symptom (e.g. difficulty with speech, diplopia), to then interpret correctly the findings you have elicited, and to make a suitable diagnosis or construct a reasonable list of differential diagnoses (e.g. histoplasmosis is not common in the UK, so do not put it first on your list of the causes of erythema nodosum!)

3. Finally, your attitude is being assessed. Do not physically injure the patient (e.g. feel for both carotid arteries at the same time; draw blood whilst using a pin to examine him for pain sensation), or cause emotional distress (e.g. use the word 'syphilis' in front of a patient, rather than a more discrete alternative such as 'luetic disease'; or bare a woman's chest at the start of your examination of the cardiovascular system, rather than when you come to palpate and auscultate the heart).

THE CANDIDATE   Dress smartly but conservatively. Do not smell of alcohol, cigarettes or curry, and make sure your hands and nails are clean. Try to appear confident and relaxed. Present your findings according to how the examiner asks for them, and in the same order in which you elicited them. Avoid abbreviations (e.g. AF, MS), and words such as 'slight', 'perhaps', 'I think', 'um' and 'er'. For example, having examined the cardiovascular system of a patient with mitral stenosis:

1. Examiner: What is the diagnosis?
   Candidate: Mitral stenosis.
2. Examiner: What abnormal signs did you find?
   Candidate: This lady has a prominent malar flush. The first heart sound is loud, and there is an opening snap, followed by a grade 3 out of 4, low-pitched, rumbling, diastolic murmur with a crescendo presystolic component. The murmur is loudest at the apex, with the patient on her left side.
3. Examiner: What are your findings?
   Candidate: This lady has a prominent malar flush, but is not breathless, cyanosed or clubbed. Her pulse rate is 84 beats per minute, and the pulse is regular and of normal volume. All her peripheral pulses are present. The jugular venous pressure is not elevated, and there is no ankle swelling. Her apex beat is in the normal position, and has a normal character. There are no palpable heart sounds or thrills. The first heart sound is loud, the second normal. In addition there is a loud opening snap, but no other added sounds and no systolic murmur. Following the opening snap there is a low-pitched, rumbling diastolic murmur, grade 3 out of 4, with a crescendo presystolic component. The murmur is loudest at the apex, with the patient turned onto her left side.

THE EXAMINERS   Examiners are given a hawk/dove index based on their own previous performances. Usually a hawk and a dove are paired together. The majority are polite and charming, but do not think you have necessarily failed if an examiner appears rude and abrupt. Never let an aggressive examiner bully you into changing your mind when you are confident of a particular diagnosis, or fluster you during your examination of the patient. On the other hand, do not argue with the examiners on a factual point even if you think you are right. Try to impress them with your own professional approach and eagerness, and listen very carefully to what they ask you to do (e.g. 'Examine this patient's heart', rather than 'Examine the cardiovascular system'), and how they want your findings presented.

THE PATIENT   Apart from introducing yourself to the patient, and obtaining his permission (e.g. 'May I examine your hand?'), only talk to him when it is necessary (e.g. 'Could you sit forward for me', whilst auscultating the base of the heart). Treat every patient with respect ('Madam/Sir'). Patient's with chronic conditions (e.g. ventricular septal defect, Holmes-Adie pupil) are used time and time again, and may have appeared in the short cases section more often than the examiner. Do not expect to be presented with very sick patients (e.g. status asthmaticus, unconscious patient).

2. Nervous system

INTRODUCTION

Patients with neurological signs are commonly used as short cases, as many of the underlying disorders are chronic and untreatable. These are often the cases most feared by the candidate. Yet the nervous system is probably the most straightforward in terms of defining the site of the lesion that results in a particular group of signs. Having determined the site, there are few pathological processes that could cause such a lesion. Such an approach to a patient with abnormal signs depends on a practical working knowledge of neuroanatomy; there are now a number of excellent textbooks designed specifically for the clinician with this approach in mind (see bibliography).

EXAMINATION OF THE CRANIAL NERVES

Patients with cranial nerve palsies are commonly used as short cases. You must be able to examine each cranial nerve quickly, be familiar with their anatomical course and be prepared with lists of the commoner causes of each palsy. Alternatively, you may be asked to examine a system (e.g. the external ocular movements). It is not likely you will be asked to examine all of the cranial nerves in one patient. There are few pet questions, other than 'where is the lesion?', and 'what is the diagnosis?' or 'what are the causes of this lesion?'.

Common causes of cranial nerve palsies
— diabetes mellitus
— tumour
— demyelination
— aneurysm
— trauma
— surgery

Rare causes
— polyarteritis
— sarcoid
— syphilis
— meningitis

OLFACTORY NERVE (I)

Very rarely asked as a short case.

Technique

Use smell bottles, and determine the distance from the nostril when the patient first detects the smell. Test each nostril separately, having checked the patient's nasal passages are clear before starting.

Typical short case: Anosmia

Common causes — following a head injury
— olfactory groove meningioma

Rare causes — frontal lobe tumour
— obstructive hydrocephalus

OPTIC NERVE (II)

Technique Two aspects:
1. Test the visual acuity: rarely asked.
Use Snellen's charts. If vision is too poor, express as ability to count fingers, detect hand movements, or distinguish light from dark. Other aspects include assessment of near vision (Jaeger's chart; newspaper), and colour vision.

Typical short case: Sudden blindness

Causes — retinal detachment
— vitreous haemorrhage (diabetes)
— temporal arteritis
— central retinal arterial or venous occlusion
— skull fracture
— eye trauma
— acute glaucoma
— toxins (methanol)

2. Test the visual fields by confrontation perimetry: often asked.
Sit opposite the patient and explain *clearly* what is expected of him. Use a 5 mm white-headed pin to compare the patient's fields with your own. The pin must be midway between you and the patient, so it subtends the same angle on both your own and the patient's retina. Test each eye separately, using the patient's hand to cover an eye. Bring the pin in along a series of arcs to a point 18–24 inches in front of the patient's eye. Be certain to define the *outer* limit of the fields. Then determine the size of the blind spot, and look for central scotoma (using a red pin). Express your findings from the patient's viewpoint.

Typical short cases **1. Temporal hemianopia**
Common. Unilateral or bilateral. Indicates chiasmal compression.

Common cause — pituitary tumour (upper fields go first)

Rare cause — craniopharyngioma (lower fields go first)

2. Homonymous hemianopia (rare)

Causes   Indicates a post-chiasmal lesion (e.g. tumour, ischaemia):
— in the optic tract: fields often incongruous
— in the internal capsule: no macular sparing
— in the occipital cortex: macular sparing. The side of the field loss is opposite to the side of the damaged cortex.

3. Quadrantic defects (rare)

Causes   — homonymous upper outer defect: lesion in the contralateral anterior temporal lobe
— homonymous lower outer defect: parietal lobe lesion. May also have visual inattention

4. Central scotoma (rare)

Common cause   — optic neuritis (e.g. multiple sclerosis)

Rare causes   — optic nerve compression: usually also have optic atrophy.
  1. Sphenoidal ridge meningioma: may also have palsies of the III, IV, V and VI nerves.
  2. Olfactory groove meningioma: may also have anosmia.
  3. Optic nerve glioma.
— toxins:
  1. Tobacco.
  2. Alcohol.
  3. Vitamin B1 or B12 deficiency.
— retinal disease involving the macula (e.g. senile macular degeneration).

5. Tunnel vision (rare)

Causes   — glaucoma
— papilloedema
— retinal disease: retinitis pigmentosa, choroidoretinitis

EXAMINATION OF THE   Common short case.
PUPILS

Technique   If possible, examine in subdued light. Use a bright light source, and *not* an ophthalmoscope. Three aspects:

1. Note size, shape and symmetry of each pupil. If the pupils are unequal, look for other clues to decide which side is abnormal (e.g. ptosis).
2. Elicit the direct and consensual light responses of each eye. Remember this reflex is relayed by the

optic nerve, and that it is a brain stem reflex so the cortex is not involved. Shine the torch from the side of the patient, making sure he does not focus on the light source, with a resulting accommodation reaction. Some normal people have slightly asymmetrical pupils which respond normally to light (physiological anisocoria). A blind eye will have a consensual but no direct light reflex.

3. Test the accommodation reflex: the convergence reflex originates in the cortex and is relayed via the oculomotor nerve, so the optic nerve is not involved.

Typical short cases	**1. Small pupil, reacting to light**
Causes	— Horner's syndrome — elderly patient

2. Small pupil, not reacting to light

Common causes	— miotics (e.g. pilocarpine) — opiates
Rare causes	— Argyll-Robertson pupil: e.g. neurosyphilis — usually bilateral, small and irregular pupils, reacting to accommodation. — pontine haemorrhage.

3. Large pupil, reacting to light

Common causes	— Holmes-Adie syndrome ('tonic pupil'): very slow reaction to light, but normal reaction to accommodation. May also have absent tendon reflexes and impaired sweating. Usually unilateral, and in women. — anxiety
Rare cause	— cortical blindness

4. Large pupil, fixed to light

Common causes	— mydriatics: atropine eye drops; poisoning with glutethimide, amphetamines or mushrooms — IIIn palsy due to compression (also marked ptosis and external ophthalmoplegia): e.g. posterior communicating artery aneurysm, prolapse of temporal lobe
Rare causes	— Argyll-Robertson pupil due to diabetes, pinealomas or brain stem encephalitis — both eyes blind: due to a lesion proximal to the lateral geniculate bodies

— compression of the tectum of the mid-brain; not, brain death

— previous trauma to the iris

5. Horner's syndrome
May be easily overlooked.

Features
1. Slightly smaller pupil; asymmetry is more obvious in a darkened room. Normal reaction to light and accommodation.
2. Ptosis: minimal or severe (when lid reaches pupil edge).
3. Enophthalmos: difficult to appreciate.
4. Impaired sweating over the forehead (dependent on the site of the lesion in the sympathetic chain).
5. Slightly bloodshot conjunctiva.
6. If congenital, the iris on the affected side remains blue-grey.

Causes
Ipsilateral damage to the sympathetic chain, at some stage along its pathway:
1. Lesions in the cavernous sinus and orbit: also cause damage to the parasympathetic fibres (so the pupil is semi-dilated, with no reaction to light), and other cranial nerves (III, IV, V or VI)
2. Lesions adjacent to the carotid artery: e.g. migraine, thrombosis, aneurysm or previous angiography
3. Lesions of the cervical sympathetic chain: e.g. sympathectomy (look for scar), previous thyroid surgery, thyroid carcinoma, cervical node metastases; or a malignancy adjacent to the jugular foramen (look for other cranial nerve palsies: IX, X, XI and XII).
4. T1 root lesion: e.g. Pancoast's (superior sulcus) tumour (look for small muscle wasting in the hands), cervical rib (young women), Klumpke's palsy, or aortic aneurysm.
5. Lesion in the centre of the cervical cord: e.g. syringobulbia, or an intraspinal tumour (glioma, ependymoma). Look for loss of reflexes, and dissociated sensory loss in the arms.
6. Lesion in the brain stem: e.g. vascular lesion, demyelination, or glioma. Look for pain and temperature loss in the opposite side of the body.
7. Others: massive unilateral cerebral infarction; congenital

Lesions 1–3 may not affect sweating at all. Lesions 4–5 affect the face, and lesion 6 may affect the entire head, neck, arms and upper trunk.

The common examination causes are syringobulbia and cervical sympathectomy.

OCULOMOTOR (III), TROCHLEAR (IV) AND ABDUCENS NERVE (VI)

These nerves control the upper eyelid, eye movements, and the pupils. Conjugate eye movements are controlled via the medial longitudinal bundle.

Technique:

Three aspects:
1. Look for ptosis (beware of contralateral exophthalmos):

Common causes
— IIIn palsy
— part of Horner's syndrome

Rare causes
— myaesthenia gravis
— progressive ocular myopathy
— dystrophia myotonica
— congenital syphilis, taboparesis
— facio-scapulo-humeral dystrophy
— (*not* VIIn lesions)

2. Test external ocular movements: first check there is no squint when the eyes are looking ahead. Test each movement separately: lateral and medial movement (lateral and medial recti); and upward and downward movement with the eye abducted (superior and inferior recti), and adducted (inferior and superior obliques, respectively). Observe each movement carefully, and ask the patient if he sees double in any direction. Test for nystagmus (see below). In a congenital squint, the angle between the longitudinal axes of the eyes remains constant on testing the eye movements, and there is no diplopia. In contrast with an acquired (paralytic) squint, the angle varies, and there is diplopia.

3. Examine the pupils: see above

Typical short cases

1. **VIn palsy:** common short case
Weakness of lateral rectus muscle. Affected eye is deviated towards the nose. Patient may compensate for this by turning the head so the normal eye is sufficiently abducted to give a single image. Images parallel and separated horizontally.

Common causes
— diabetes
— atherosclerosis (or idiopathic)
— raised intracranial pressure (false localising sign)

Rare causes
See Table 2.1

2. **IVn palsy:** very rare short case
Weakness of superior oblique muscle. Failure of downward movement when the eye is adducted. Compensated for by tilting the head slightly away from the side of the affected eye. Subtle diplopia: two images at an angle.

Site of lesion	Structure involved	Adjacent structures	Causes
Brain stem	Nerve nuclei and nerve exit	V, VIIn Long tracts Sympathetic fibres Cerebellar connections Medial longitudinal bundle	Multiple sclerosis Vascular lesion Tumours — intrinsic or extrinsic Wernicke's encephalopathy
Skull base	Nerves	Pituitary Circle of Willis Basilar artery Posterior cerebral artery Petrous temporal bone (VIn) Sphenoidal ridge Meninges and subarachnoid space	Tumours Aneurysms (IIIn and post. comm. A) Raised intracranial pressure (VIn) Malignant infiltration Parasellar lesions Meningitis (including TB, syphilis, carcinoma)
Cavernous sinus	Nerves	Paranasal sinuses Va	Tumours Granulomas Trauma
Orbit	Nerves Neuromuscular junction Extraocular ms.	Eyeball, extraocular ms. and connective tissue Optic nerve	Tumours Granulomas Trauma Myaesthenia gravis Thyrotoxicosis
Nerve			Isolated lesion (e.g. diabetes, hypertension, temporal arteritis). Part of a generalised neuropathy (eg diabetes, Gullain-Barré syndrome).

Table 2.1 Causes of III, IV or VI nerve palsies

Most apparent to the patient on descending a staircase, or reading a newspaper.

Causes: See Table 2.1

3. IIIn palsy: rare short case
May be complete or partial.

Complete Total paralysis of the eyelid. Lift the lid, and the eye is seen to be deviated outwards (action of lateral rectus muscle), and downwards (superior oblique). Severe diplopia in all directions, except on lateral gaze to the side of the lesion (intact lateral rectus). You need to confirm:
1. IVn is intact: look for intorsion of the affected eye on attempting to look down.
2. VIn is intact: test lateral gaze in the affected eye, and note disappearance of diplopia.
   Pupil will either be normal (suggesting a medical cause for the palsy), or dilated and fixed to light (suggests a surgical cause, i.e. a compressive lesion).

Common causes	— diabetes — raised intracranial pressure
Rare causes	See Table 2.1
Partial	Where only parts of the IIIn nucleus are affected, resulting in paresis of individual orbital muscles.

'This man has diplopia. Examine him': common short case

The possibilities are:

1. This is due to a lesion of one or more of the III, IV or VI nerves. This can usually be detected by observation of the external ocular movements. If not:
   a. Ask the patient in which direction the diplopia is worse: diplopia is maximum when looking in the direction of action of the paralysed muscle.
   b. Ask whether the images are parallel to each other (lateral rectus weakness), or at an angle (superior oblique weakness).
   c. Cover each eye in turn and ask which image disappears: the outer image arises from the paralysed eye.

2. The muscle itself is the cause:

Common cause	— thyrotoxicosis (lateral or superior rectus)
Rare causes	— myaesthenia gravis (varying eye signs, fatiguable eye movements) — dystrophia myotonica

3. There is disruption of the conjugate eye movement mechanism.

Common cause	— multiple sclerosis. Classical internuclear ophthalmoplegia: weakness of *ad*ducting eye, and nystagmus in the *ab*ducting eye.
Rare cause	— Wernicke's encephalopathy. Variable defect in conjugate gaze, with weakness of lateral rectus, and horizontal and/or vertical nystagmus.

NYSTAGMUS

This is due either to a weakness in maintaining conjugate eye deviation, or to an imbalance in the postural control of eye movements. Remember, the tendency of the deviated eye to move back to the control position (slow component) is the pathological component. But it is the fast flick (fast component) to regain the original position that is recorded as the direction of nystagmus.

'This man has nystagmus. Examine him': rare short case

1. Look for nystagmus at rest.
2. Determine which eye movements exacerbate or provoke nystagmus ('on upward, downward or lateral gaze'). Coarse nystagmoid jerks may be provoked in

a normal patient if asked to follow an object too far to the side, or if that object is too close.

3. Determine the direction of the fast component ('horizontal, vertical or rotatory'). Horizontal nystagmus on vertical gaze is not vertical nystagmus.
4. Describe the nystagmus as fine or coarse
5. Determine whether the nystagmus is sustained (i.e. continues for the duration of your examination), or not sustained.

Causes

1. *Congenital* (rare): dramatic. Non-stop, side-to-side, pendular movements of the eyes; exaggerated on gazing in any direction. Similar nystagmus may be seen in coal-miners, and with certain retinal diseases.

2. *Vestibular disease*: lesion affecting VIIIn or the semicircular canals (peripheral), or the VIIIn nucleus (central). Usually associated with deafness, vertigo or tinnitus. Greater on looking away from the side of the destructive lesion.
   a. Peripheral lesion: features:
      — horizontal or rotatory nystagmus
      — unidirectional and conjugate nystagmus
      — accompanied by vertigo
      — early central compensation (3–4 weeks)
      — enhanced by loss of visual fixation

Common causes
   — viral labyrinthitis
   — Ménière's disease

Rare causes
   — acute alcoholism
   — middle ear disease
   — surgery.

   b. Central lesion: features:
      — nystagmus may be vertical
      — multidirectional and dysconjugate nystagmus
      — often no vertigo
      — nystagmus persists
      — little affected by loss of visual fixation

Common cause
   — multiple sclerosis

Rare causes
   — basilar artery ischaemia
   — syringobulbia
   — glioma

3. *Cerebellar disease*: lateral lobe lesions (may be absent in midline lesions and cerebellar degenerative disease). Greater on looking *towards* the damaged side. Otherwise similar features to central vestibular lesions.

Common cause — multiple sclerosis

Rare causes — hereditary ataxias
— vascular disease
— tumour

4. *Ataxic nystagmus*: nystagmus greater in the *ab*ducting eye than the *ad*ducting one (classical internuclear ophthalmoplegia); if bilateral, pathognomonic of multiple sclerosis.

5. *Drugs*: sedatives (barbiturates), anticonvulsants (phenytoin, carbamazepine), or alcohol.

TRIGEMINAL NERVE (V)   Rare short case.

Technique   Three aspects:
1. Sensory: Va supplies the conjunctiva, lacrimal gland, upper eyelids, forehead, and scalp up to the vertex. Vb supplies the cheek, nose, upper lip and teeth, roof of the mouth and most of the soft palate. Vc supplies the lower part of the face, ear, lower lip and teeth, and the anterior two-thirds of the tongue.
2. Motor: 'Clench your teeth': feel masseter and temporalis muscles. 'Open your mouth and keep it open', as you try to close it by pushing the lower jaw up: pterygoids (jaw will deviate towards the weak muscle). (Remember: does *not* supply the muscles of facial expression).
3. Reflexes: corneal reflex (earliest sign of Vn damage), and jaw jerk.

Causes of Vn palsy   — cerebellopontine angle lesions (may have evidence of VII or VIIIn lesion, ipsilateral cerebellar signs, and contralateral long tract signs in the limbs (due to pontine compression)): VIIIn tumour, meningioma, cholesteatoma, basilar artery aneurysm, or carcinoma (nasopharyngeal, or metastases)
— Vn tumour
— multiple sclerosis
— herpes zoster, Vn sensory neuropathy, dystrophia myotonica

FACIAL NERVE (VII)   Common short case.

Technique   Three aspects (though only expected to test the first in a short case):

1. Motor supply to the muscles of facial expression. Look for facial asymmetry at rest. Test:
   a. frontalis muscle: ability to wrinkle forehead and lift eyebrows ('look up at the ceiling').

    b. ability to shut eyes tightly: try to forcibly open the eyes.

    c. ability to smile, show his teeth (an upper motor neurone lesion may be more obvious in a spontaneous than in a voluntary movement).

2. Sensation: taste of anterior two-thirds of the tongue (chorda tympani n.).

3. Secretomotor: lacrimation (Schirmer's test). Relayed via the greater superficial petrosal nerve.

Typical short cases

1. Upper motor neurone facial weakness
Weakness of the lower face with normal eye closure and forehead wrinkling.

Causes
— cerebrovascular accident
— cerebral tumour

2. Lower motor neurone facial weakness
All muscles affected. During recovery, restoration of the frontalis and orbicularis oculi muscles occurs before those of the lower face.

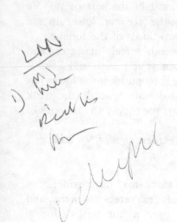

Causes

1. Intracranial:
— brain stem lesion (infarction, demyelination)
— cerebellopontine angle lesion
— VIIn neuroma or neurofibroma

2. During passage through temporal bone:
— fracture
— surgical procedure
— otitis media
— middle ear carcinoma
— Ramsey-Hunt syndrome (herpes zoster: look for vesicles around external auditory meatus)

3. Extracranial:
— parotid tumour
— trauma

4. General conditions:

Common
— idiopathic (Bell's palsy)
— diabetes mellitus
— hypertension

Rare
— sarcoid
— infectious mononucleosis
— connective tissue disease
— Melkersson's syndrome (facial oedema, fissured tongue)
— dystrophia myotonica

AUDITORY NERVE (VIII)

Very rare short case.
Three aspects:
1. Hearing: determine the distance from each ear that the patient can hear whispered words or a wristwatch ticking.
2. Weber's test: tuning fork is heard in the normal ear in perceptive deafness.
3. Rinne's test: normally positive (i.e. air conduction louder than bone). Preferably use a 512 Hz tuning fork.

Typical short case: Deafness

Causes:

1. Conductive deafness:
— wax
— otitis media
— otosclerosis (blue sclerae)
2. Perceptive deafness:
— trauma
— infection (mumps, flu, congenital rubella)
— toxins: aspirin, streptomycin
— presbyacusis
— VIIIn tumour

'This patient has vertigo. Examine him': very rare short case

Look for:
1. Hearing loss: conductive or perceptive deafness.
2. Nystagmus.

Causes

— peripheral vestibular (labyrinthine) disorders: e.g. Ménière's disease, benign paroxysmal positional vertigo, migraine
— central vestibular disorders: e.g. multiple sclerosis, tumour, infarction, transient ischaemic attack
— external influences on the vestibular system: e.g. drugs (alcohol; phenytoin, aspirin, streptomycin), anaemia, viruses (vestibular neuronitis), syphilis

GLOSSOPHARYNGEAL NERVE (IX)

Very rarely asked. Conveys sensation from the palate and posterior pharyngeal wall (sensory part of the gag reflex), and taste from the posterior third of the tongue. Also provides the motor supply to stylopharyngeus muscle, which cannot be assessed clinically.

VAGUS NERVE (X)

Very rarely asked. Motor supply to the palate and vocal cords. Weakness results in nasal speech, nasal regurgitation of food, and bovine cough. When asked to say 'Aah', the paralysed side of the palate and uvula moves across to the intact side.

SPINAL ACCESSORY NERVE (XI)

Very rarely asked. Motor supply to sternomastoid ('put your chin over your left (or right) shoulder', whilst you resist the movement and palpate the right (or left)

muscle), and upper part of trapezius muscle ('shrug your shoulders', whilst you push them down).

HYPOGLOSSAL NERVE (XII)   Rarely asked. Motor supply to the tongue. 'Put out your tongue': will deviate toward the weaker side. Look for wasting and fasciculation of the weaker side (lower motor neurone lesion). 'Move your tongue from side to side'.

Typical short cases
1. Bulbar palsy: rare short case
Nasal speech, flaccid fasciculating tongue, normal or absent jaw jerk: due to bilateral lower motor neurone lesions of IX, X, and XII nerves.

Causes
— motor neurone disease
— polio
— syringobulbia
— Guillain-Barré syndrome

2. Pseudobulbar palsy: rare short case
'Donald Duck' speech, spastic tongue, increased jaw jerk, labile emotions, and bilateral pyramidal signs in the limbs: due to bilateral upper motor neurone lesions of IX, X and XII nerves.

Causes
— bilateral internal capsule cerebrovascular accidents
— multiple sclerosis

3. Unilateral IX, X, XI or XIIn palsies: very rare

Causes
— lesions in or around the jugular foramen, either inside the skull (look for features of brain stem compression) or outside (look for Horner's syndrome): e.g. neurinomas, meningioma, metastatic deposit
— carotid body tumours: IXn, Xn

EXAMINATION OF THE EYES   Patients with abnormal eye signs are very common short cases. Such a finding may lead on to being asked to examine other systems to determine the cause. You must, therefore, be prepared with lists of the known associations of each abnormal eye sign.

'EXAMINE THIS MAN'S EYES'

Technique   This should include the following:

1. Look for proptosis. If suspicious, stand behind the patient, look down the front of his face and compare the prominence of each eye; express the difference in millimetres. Beware of *en*ophthalmos

Common causes
— thyrotoxicosis (may be unilateral)
— orbital tumours (primary or secondary)

Rare causes — carotico-cavernous fistula
— orbital cellulitis
— carotid sinus thrombosis
— sphenoidal ridge meningioma

2. Look at the eyelids for:
   a. xanthelasmata

Common causes — diabetes
— hyperlipidaemia
— hypothyroidism

Rare cause — primary biliary cirrhosis

   b. ptosis
   c. lid retraction: thyrotoxicosis
   d. infections (stye), rodent ulcer, ectropion,
      entropion (all rare)
   e. violaceous rash: dermatomyositis
   f. swelling (very rare)

Causes — nephrotic syndrome
— contact dermatitis (antibiotic eyedrops, cosmetics:
  eczema of periorbital skin)
— hereditary angioedema (C1 esterase deficiency)
— rosacea

3. Look at the cornea and sclera for:
   a. arcus senilis: maximum at 6 and 12 o'clock.

Causes — old age
— hyperlipidaemia

   b. Calcification: maximum at 3 and 9 o'clock (rare).

Cause — hypercalcaemia

   c. Kayser-Fleischer rings: Wilson's disease (rare).
   d. Conjunctivitis, corneal graft, interstitial keratitis
      (all rare).
   e. Anaemia, jaundice, blue sclerae (osteogenesis
      imperfecta, Ehlers-Danlos syndrome).
4. Test the optic nerve: visual acuity, and visual fields
   to confrontation.
5. Test the external ocular movements, noting the presence or absence of a squint, or nystagmus.
6. Test the pupillary reflexes.
7. With the ophthalmoscope, look at the:
   a. Iris and anterior chamber: e.g. iritis, glaucoma
      (rare).
   b. Lens: cataract or opacities.

Common causes — senility
— diabetes
— trauma

Rare causes   — congenital (Down's syndrome, dystrophia myotonica)
— hypoparathyroidism
— irradiation
— drugs (steroids, chloroquine)

c. Fundus.

EXAMINATION OF THE FUNDUS   Almost every candidate is asked to examine a fundus in the short cases section. Take your own ophthalmoscope, or one whose use you are familiar with, as the one preferred by the examiner may not be ideal.

Technique   Ask the patient to focus on a specific distant object ('look at those flowers'). Look at the patient's *right* eye, from his *right* side, using your own *right* eye with the ophthalmoscope in your *right* hand, and vice versa. Start looking through the eyepiece at the patient's eye from a distance, to test for the red reflex (absent with a false eye, cataract, or retinal tumour). Then bring the ophthalmoscope up to the eye, inspecting the iris, lens and then retina. Comment on the disc, vessels and retina. Remeber that myopic patients have deep optic cups and temporal pallor (?optic atrophy), whilst hypermetropic discs look smaller and pinker, and have ill-defined margins (?early papilloedema).

Typical short cases   Be familiar with the rare as well as the common fundal abnormalities, if not by experience at the bedside, then by looking at photographs in textbooks (see bibliography).

1. Hypertensive fundus: very common short case

Features   Keith, Wagener and Barber classification:

Grade 1: diffuse or segmental arteriolar narrowing with thickened walls give a heightened reflex ('silver-wiring').
Grade 2: nipping of veins at points of arterial crossing (A-V nipping).
Grade 3: flame-shaped haemorrhages and soft exudates (retinal microinfarctions: 'cotton-wool' spots). Deeper waxy exudates ('hard exudates').
Grade 4: oedema of the optic disc.

2. Diabetic fundus: very common short case

Features   1. 'Background retinopathy': microaneurysms, dot and blot haemorrhages, vitreous haemorrhages, venous looping and beading, and hard exudates.
2. 'Proliferative retinopathy'; cotton-wool spots, new vessel formation, fibrous patches, and rubeosis of the iris. Photocoagulation changes: peripherally placed pigmented scars ('moon-craters').

3. Optic atrophy: common short case

Features — Primary: very pale disc with distinct lamina cribrosa; may be simulated by a temporal pigment rim.
Secondary: flat, grey-white disc with indistinct edges.

Common causes
— after optic neuritis (multiple sclerosis)
— optic nerve compression (with papilloedema on the opposite side: Foster Kennedy syndrome)
— trauma or ischaemia

Rare causes
— following papilloedema (secondary)
— glaucoma
— toxins (tobacco, methanol)
— B1 or B12 deficiency
— neurosyphilis
— hereditary (Leber's disease)

4. Papilloedema: rare short case

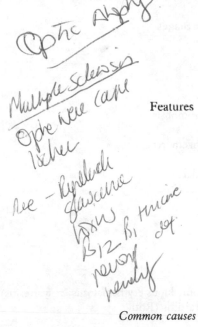

Features — Large blind spot, with normal acuity. Sequence of changes:
1. Increase in venous calibre and tortuosity, and loss of venous pulsation.
2. Pink optic cup, lamina cribrosa cannot be seen, indistinct nasal edge, and arteriovenous nipping.
3. Swollen optic cup, with blurring of the temporal margin.
4. Whole disc swollen; origins of vessels cannot be seen. Flame-shaped haemorrhages.
Appearances may be simulated by optic neuritis (central scotoma, poor visual acuity, pain on eye movements), and myelinated nerve fibres.

Common causes
— raised intracranial pressure
— malignant (grade 4) hypertension

Rare causes
— raised CSF protein (e.g. Guillain-Barré syndrome)
— metabolic disorders (e.g. hypercapnia)
— circulatory disorders (e.g. macroglobulinaemia, polycythaemia)

5. Choroidoretinitis: rare short case

Features — Irregular areas of exposed white sclera with dark patches of proliferated retinal pigment epithelium.

Common causes
— idiopathic
— toxoplasmosis
— diabetes
— sarcoid

Rare causes	— toxocara — tuberculosis — syphilis

6. Retinitis pigmentosa: rare

Features	Spider-like nets of pigment at the periphery of the retina.
Causes	— isolated abnormality — Refsum's disease (deafness, ataxia, peripheral neuropathy and hypertrophied nerves) — Laurence-Moon-Biedl syndrome (polydactyly, obesity, hypogonadism, mental retardation)

7. Retinal haemorrhages

Common causes	— hypertension — diabetes
Rare causes	— papilloedema — retinal vein thrombosis — arteritis — subarachnoid haemorrhage — anaemia — bleeding disorder — infective endocarditis

8. Soft exudates

Common causes	— hypertension — diabetes
Rare causes	— vasculitis (systemic lupus erythematosus, polyarteritis) — infective endocarditis (Roth's spots)

EXAMINATION OF THE PERIPHERAL NERVOUS SYSTEM

Patients with lesions of the peripheral nervous system are commonly used as short cases. The abnormalities seen will either be in isolation (e.g. Klumpke's palsy), or as part of a more generalised disorder (e.g. Friedreich's ataxia). The site of the lesion may be either central (cortex, brain stem, or spinal cord) or peripheral (spinal root, trunk, nerve, neuromuscular junction, or muscle).

You are only likely to be asked to perform a neurological examination of one limb, or a pair of limbs, or to observe a gait or involuntary movement. When asked simply to examine a foot or hand, remember that the nervous system is only part of the examination.

Technique   Four aspects to remember:

1. Motor system
2. Spinal reflexes
3. Sensory system
4. Coordination

EXAMINE THE MOTOR SYSTEM

Inspection   Look specifically for:
— involuntary movements
— muscle fasciculation: physiological (after exertion) or pathological (motor neurone disease; lower motor neurone disorders)
— muscle wasting or hypertrophy: note its distribution
— abnormal posture or contracture: e.g. claw hand, foot drop, pes cavus

Palpation   Assess muscle tone.

Hypertonia   May be due to:

1. Corticospinal tract lesion (spasticity): e.g. in hemiplegia, the spasticity predominantly affects one or other of the opposing muscle groups (upper limb flexors, lower limb extensors), and shows a 'clasp-knife' effect (i.e. the maximum resistance is at the outset of the passive movement).
2. Extrapyramidal disease (rigidity): e.g. in Parkinsonism, rigidity is present to an equal extent in opposing muscle groups, and is uniform throughout the whole range of movement at a joint ('cogwheel': interrupted, or 'leadpipe': smooth character).
3. Dystrophia myotonica and myotonia congenita: hypertonia is the result of prolongation of a voluntary muscular contraction.

Hypotonia   May be due to:

1. Lower motor neurone lesion
2. A lesion of the sensory afferents: e.g. tabes dorsalis
3. Cerebellar disease
4. Spinal shock

Power   Assess muscle power in groups, and record your findings according to the MRC scale:

0   no contraction
1   flicker or trace of contraction
2   active movement, with gravity eliminated

3   active movement, against gravity
4   active movement, against gravity and resistance
5   normal power

Patterns of motor loss in the limbs

1. Upper motor neurone (pyramidal) lesion

Features

1. Reduced or absent power, with little wasting. The weakness is more marked in the upper limb extensors, and lower limb flexors.
2. Spasticity: sustained ankle clonus.
3. Extensor plantar responses, absent superficial abdominal reflexes.
4. Exaggerated tendon reflexes.

Causes

Lesions in:
1. Cerebral cortex, subcortical area, or internal capsule: e.g.
— vascular lesions
— neoplasms
2. Brain stem: e.g.
— demyelination
— vascular lesions
— neoplasms
3. Spinal cord: e.g.
— demyelination
— compression
— motor neurone disease (lower limbs)
— subacute combined degeneration (lower limbs)
— Friedreich's ataxia (lower limbs)
— tabes dorsalis (lower limbs)
— syringomyelia (lower limbs)

2. Lower motor neurone lesion

Features

1. Marked muscle wasting, with reduced or absent power.
2. Hypotonia.
3. Absent tendon reflexes and plantar responses.

Causes

— lesions involving the anterior horn cells in the spinal cord: e.g. motor neurone disease, polio
— peripheral neuropathy

3. Muscle or muscle end plate lesion

Features

Weakness, with or without wasting, in a distribution which does not correspond with a root or nerve supply.

Causes

— myopathies: symmetrical wasting with weakness
— myaesthenia gravis: striking increase in weakness on fatigue. Signs are usually a late and minor feature.

No wasting. Normal reflexes. Variable ptosis, or extraocular or facial muscle weakness.
— myaesthenic syndrome (Eaton-Lambert syndrome): decrease in weakness on fatigue, usually affecting the proximal muscles of the pelvic and shoulder girdles. Associated with oat-cell bronchial carcinoma.

TEST THE SPINAL REFLEXES   1. Deep or tendon reflexes: if absent, test again with reinforcement (Jendrassek manoeuvre). Remember the pendular reflex in cerebellar disease, and the sustained contraction in myxoedema.
2. Superficial or cutaneous reflexes: you are only likely to be asked to examine the plantar response, or, rarely, the abdominal reflexes (test all four quadrants).

Diminution or absence of tendon reflexes

Common causes   — peripheral neuropathy: distal reflexes affected more than proximal
— other lower motor neurone lesions
— old age: ankle jerks commonly absent
— diabetes mellitus: may have depressed knee and ankle jerks in the absence of other signs or peripheral neuropathy
— Holmes-Adie syndrome: absent leg reflexes, and 'tonic pupils'
— syringomyelia

Absent knee and ankle jerks, with extensor plantar response

Causes   — subacute combined degeneration of the cord
— taboparesis
— Friedreich's ataxia
— motor neurone disease
— diabetic amyotrophy

EXAMINE THE SENSORY SYSTEM   Be familiar with the cutaneous areas of distribution of the spinal segments (dermatomes):

C2   back of head, angle of jaw
C3   neck
C4   front and back of upper chest
C5–T2 upper limb
T4   chest, at level of the nipples (men)
T7   chest, at the level of the lower ribs
T10   abdomen, at the level of the umbilicus
L1   inguinal region
L2–S2 lower limb
S3–4   external genitalia, buttocks

Technique

Four main groups of modalities:

1. Tactile sensation: accurate light touch (tip of finger, fine wisp of cotton wool), and two-point discrimination (unlikely to be asked in a short case). Impulses carried in the ipsilateral dorsal columns of the spinal cord.
2. Joint position sense: dorsal columns.
3. Vibration sense: use a 128 Hz tuning fork, and yourself as a control. Originally thought to be carried in the dorsal column, but probably carried in several pathways.
4. Pain and temperature sensation: contralateral spinothalamic tract.

Patterns of sensory loss in the limbs

1. Parietal lobe lesion (rare short case): poor two-point discrimination, astereognosis, agraphaesthesia and sensory inattention.
2. Spinal cord lesion (rare):
   a. Spinothalamic loss, without dorsal column loss ('dissociated sensory loss'): e.g. syringomyelia (loss in both arms), cord hemisection (Brown-Séquard syndrome: contralateral spinothalamic and ipsilateral dorsal column loss).
   b. Dorsal column loss alone: e.g. subacute combined degeneration, tabes dorsalis.
3. Peripheral sensory neuropathy (common): symmetrical loss of all modalities ('glove and stocking').
4. Lesions of spinal nerve roots or individual peripheral nerves (common).

TEST COORDINATION

Incoordination may be due to sensory loss (worse when the patient closes his eyes), to lesions involving the cerebellum or its connections, or to muscle weakness.

NEUROLOGICAL EXAMINATION OF THE UPPER LIMB

Common short case.

1. Examine the motor system

Inspection

Quickly look for any obvious muscle wasting (note its distribution), fasciculation, involuntary movement, abnormal posture, or trophic changes.

Palpation

Assess muscle tone at the elbow and/or wrist joint. In a pyramidal lesion, the spasticity predominantly affects the flexors of the upper limb.

Test muscle power

Use a systematic approach. Assess power in muscle groups, working from the shoulder downwards (or vice versa), remembering that for each of the basic movements of the arm there is a single root value and peripheral nerve supply (Table 2.2).

Joint	Movement	Root	Nerve	Muscle
Shoulder	Abduction: first 90°	C5	Suprascapular	Supraspinatus
	second 90°	C5	Axillary	Deltoid
	Adduction	C7	Latissimus dorsi	Latiss. dorsi
				Pectoralis major
	External rotation	C5	Suprascapular	Infraspinatus
	Internal rotation	C5	Subscapular	Subscapularis
				Teres minor
Elbow	Flexion, when fully	C5	Musculocutaneous	Biceps
	supinated			Brachialis
	Flexion, when half supinated	C6	Radial	Brachioradialis
	Extension	C7	Radial	Triceps
	Supination	C6	Radial	Supinator
	Pronation	C6	Median	Pronator teres
				Quadratus
Wrist	Flexion	C7,8	Median	Forearm flexors
			Ulnar	Flexor carpi ulnaris
	Extension	C7	Radial	Forearm extensors
Thumb	Abduction	T1	Median	Abductor pollicis brevis
	Pinching movement	C8	Anterior	Long flexor of thumb and index
			interosseous	finger
Finger	Flexion: index and middle	C8	Median	Flexor digitorum profundus
	ring and little	C8	Ulnar	
	Extension	C8	Radial	Finger extensors
	Abduction	T1	Ulnar	Interossei and abductor digiti
				minimi

Table 2.2 Motor supply of the upper limb

1. Ask the patient to hold his arms outstretched in front of him, and to then close his eyes. This is useful as a screen for:
   a. Weakness of shoulder abduction (C5): the arm will drift downwards.
   b. Cerebellar lesion: the arm on the affected side tends to hyperpronate, and to rise above the other arm.
   c. Loss of joint position sense: the affected arm tends to drift away from the other (equivalent of Romberg's test in the legs).
2. As a minimum, without the benefit of asking the patient which muscles are weak, test:

	Root supply	nerve supply
Shoulder abduction	C5	axillary, supra-scapular
Elbow flexion (with forearm half supinated)	C6	radial
Wrist extension	C7	radial
Finger flexion at the distal inter-phalangeal joint of the index finger	C8	median
Thumb opposition	C8	median
Finger abduction	T1	ulnar

The ability to grip involves several muscle groups, and thus several roots and nerves; there is therefore no diagnostic value in testing grip strength when defining root and nerve lesions.

2. Test the reflexes
Each deep tendon reflex of the arm also has a root value and a peripheral nerve value.

	Root supply	Nerve supply
Biceps	C5	musculocutaneous
Supinator	C6	radial
Triceps	C7	radial
Finger flexion (index, middle)	C8	median

3. Examine the sensory system
Sensory signs are far less reliable than motor findings when evaluating root and nerve lesion (Table 2.3), due to overlapping of territories by other nerves. As a minimum, test for light touch and pain sensation in each of the dermatomes, and check vibration and joint position sense on a finger.

Root/nerve lesion	Distribution
C5	Lateral border of the upper arm
C6	Lateral forearm, including thumb
C7	Middle fingers
C8	Medial forearm, including little finger
T1	Axilla down to the olecranon
Axillary	Small area over the deltoid muscle
Musculocutaneous	Lateral forearm
Radial	Dorsum of thumb and index finger or may be none
Ulnar	Medial palm; little and medial half of ring finger
Median	Lateral palm, and lateral $3\frac{1}{2}$ digits

Table 2.3   Sensory loss in the upper limb

4. Test coordination
Finger–nose testing, with the eyes open and then closed. Look for intention tremor, or past pointing. Other cerebellar signs are described on page 34.

Typical short cases

1. Individual peripheral nerve lesions
Most commonly the result of pressure neuropathy, but may be part of a mononeuritis multiplex (diabetes, polyarteritis, leprosy, sarcoid, or systemic lupus erythematosus).

Median nerve: common short case

Common cause — Carpal tunnel syndrome, which occurs in:
— middle-aged women
— arthritis or after fractures involving the wrist joint
— pregnancy
— myxoedema, acromegaly, nephrotic syndrome, amyloidosis

Features — hollowing of the outer half of the thenar eminence
— weakness of abduction and opposition of the thumb; no weakness of the other hand muscles
— variable sensory loss, ranging from no loss at all to total loss of sensation over the lateral $3\frac{1}{2}$ digits (the palm escapes because the palmar branch of the median nerve lies superficial to the flexor retinaculum)
— Tinel's sign: tingling in the appropriate distribution produced by a sharp tap over the carpal ligament

Rare cause — Lesion of the anterior interosseous nerve (e.g. dislocation of the elbows, forearm fracture) results in additional weakness of the long flexors of the thumb and index finger.

Ulnar nerve: rare short case

Common cause — Lesion in the neighbourhood of the elbow (repeated trauma, previous fracture, or arthritis).

Features — 1. Wasting of the muscles in the hypothenar eminence, interosseous spaces, and ulnar half of the thenar eminence. The fingers are hyperextentded at the MCP joint, and flexed at the IP joints: this is most marked in the ring and little fingers (as the lumbricals of the index and middle fingers are supplied by the median nerve): 'claw hand' or 'papal blessing' sign.
2. Weakness of all the intrinsic hand muscles, except abductor pollicis brevis and opponens pollicis. When examining finger abduction or adduction, keep the patient's palm pressed against a flat surface to prevent the long finger extensors and flexors acting as abductors and adductors.
3. Weakness of the ulnar half of flexor digitorum profundus (flexes the little and ring fingers at the distal interphalangeal joint), and flexor carpi ulnaris (hand deviates to the radial side on flexion of the wrist against gravity).
4. Variable sensory loss, ranging from no loss at all to anaesthesia of the medial $1\frac{1}{2}$ digits and the ulnar border of the palm.

Rare cause   Lesion in the wrist: pressure neuropathy of the deep branch, due to repeated trauma to the heel of the hand (e.g. use of a screwdriver). The wasting and weakness is limited to the interossei (finger abduction and adduction) and adductors to the thumb, and there is no sensory loss.   ·

Wasting of the intrinsic muscles of the hand

Causes   — rheumatoid arthritis: characteristic joint stigmata
— ulnar nerve lesion
— peripheral neuropathy
— injury to the lower part of the brachial plexus: e.g. Klumpke palsy, Pancoast's tumour, or cervical rib
— T1 root lesion: wasting and weakness of *all* the intrinsic hand muscles (cf ulnar nerve palsy): e.g. cervical spondylosis
— cord disease at C8, T1: e.g. syringomyelia, motor neurone disease, spinal tumour or cord compression,
— Charcot-Marie-Tooth disease (rare feature)

Radial nerve: very rare short case

Features   Vulnerable to pressure at three sites:
1. In the axilla: e.g. incorrect use of a crutch. Results in wrist-drop, finger-drop (remember the long extensors act only at the metacarpophalangeal joints), and weakness of elbow extension (triceps) and flexion (of half-supinated forearm: brachioradialis). Absent triceps reflex. Usually no sensory loss.
2. In the spiral groove of the humerus: e.g. midshaft fracture, 'Saturday-night palsy'. As in (1), but spares the triceps, so triceps reflex is present.
3. Damage to the posterior interosseus nerve as it passes through the supinator muscle: e.g. excessive use of a screwdriver. Results in weakness of extension of the wrist, thumb and index finger.

Remember: (a) A C6 lesion results in weakness of elbow flexion in both the fully supinated (biceps) and half-supinated forearm (brachioradialis); radial nerve lesions only affect brachioradialis. (b) A C7 lesion results in weakness of shoulder adduction, elbow extension and wrist extension and flexion; radial nerve lesions do not affect shoulder adduction or wrist flexion, and also weaken elbow flexion and supination.

Other nerve lesions: very rare short cases

1. Long thoracic nerve: winging of the scapula, with inability to raise the arm forwards and upwards (weakness of serratus anterior).

2. Axillary nerve: wasting and weakness of the deltoid muscle (second 90° of shoulder abduction), with overlying sensory loss. A C5 root lesion will weaken all 180° of shoulder abduction.

2. Brachial plexus lesions
Rare short cases, but used as 'spot diagnoses'.

Upper plexus (Erb-Duchenne palsy)   Avulsion of C5 and C6 roots.

Features   The limb hangs at the side, with the elbow extended and the forearm pronated ('Porter's tip' position).

Causes   — birth injury (affected limb is often smaller than the other side)
— fall

Lower plexus   C8 and T1 roots

Features   Wasting and weakness of all the intrinsic hand muscles ('claw hand'), and of the long flexors and extensors of the fingers.

Causes   — Dejerine-Klumpke type of birth palsy, trauma
— cervical rib: young women. May also have an ipsilateral Horner's syndrome, vascular signs (unequal radial pulses, gangrene) or a palpable rib in the neck
— Pancoast's tumour: may also have Horner's syndrome

3. Spinal root lesions
Rare short cases.

Cervical spondylosis

Features   The result of (1) root compression: usually affects C5, 6 or 7; (2) compressive cervical myelopathy (less common): progressive spastic paraplegia.
a. Usually only slight weakness of the muscles innervated by the affected spinal roots.
b. Some loss of light touch and pin-prick within the affected dermatomes.
c. Absent or depressed tendon reflexes may help localise the spinal lesion: e.g. absent biceps (C5) and supinator (C6) jerks with an exaggerated triceps jerk is diagnostic of cervical spondylosis with C5–6 root and C7 cord compression.

Other causes: very rare short cases   — inflammatory or neoplastic lesions involving the spinal meninges
— vertebral body collapse: Paget's, infection, neoplasms

NEUROLOGICAL
EXAMINATION OF THE
LOWER LIMB

Less commonly asked in a short case than the upper limb.

1. Examine the motor system

Inspection   Look particularly for:
1. Wasting: more difficult to detect than in the upper limb.
2. Abnormal shape or posture: e.g. foot drop, pes cavus, or 'inverted champagne bottles' (Charcot-Marie-Tooth disease).
3. Hypertrophied calves (Duchenne dystrophy), fasciculation, or trophic changes.

Palpation   Assess muscle tone, and test for ankle clonus. In a pyramidal lesion, the spasticity predominantly affects the extensors of the lower limb.

Joint	Movement	Root	Nerve	Muscle
Hip	Flexion	L23	Femoral	Iliacus
			Psoas	Psoas
	Extension	L45	Inferior gluteal	Gluteus maximus
	Abduction	L45	Superior gluteal	Gluteus medius and minimus
	Abduction	L234	Femoral	Quadriceps
Knee	Flexion	L5S1	Tibial, peroneal	Hamstrings
	Extension	L234	Femoral	Quadriceps
Foot	Plantarflexion	S12	Tibial	Gastrocnemii
				Tibialis posterior
	Dorsiflexion	L45	Peroneal	Tibialis anterior
				Long extensors
				Peroneus tertius
				Extensor digitorum brevis
	Inversion	L4	Tibial, peroneal	Tibialis anterior and posterior
	Eversion	S1	Peroneal	Peroneus longus and brevis
				Extensor digitorum brevis

Table 2.4   Motor supply of the lower limb

Test power in muscle groups   Most muscles have a nerve supply derived from two roots (Table 2.4) so weakness is often difficult to detect in individual root lesions. As a minimum test:

	Root supply	Nerve supply
Hip flexion	L23	psoas, femoral
Knee extension	L(2)34	femoral
Foot dorsiflexion	L45	peroneal
Knee flexion	L5S1	tibial, peroneal
Foot plantarflexion	S12	tibial

2. Test the reflexes

a. Tendon:

	Root supply	Nerve supply
Knee	L4	femoral
Ankle	S1	tibial

b. Superficial: plantar response. It is the first movement of the big toe which is recorded. A Babinski response is an extensor plantar response; there is no such thing as a 'negative Babinski'.

Root/nerve lesion	Distribution
L2	Across upper thigh, or may be none
L3	Across lower thigh, or may be none
L4	Medial side of leg
L5	Dorsum of foot, big toe, sole
S1	Behind lateral malleolus, back of calf
Obturator	Medial surface of thigh: often none
Femoral	Anteromedial surface of thigh and leg to the medial malleolus
Peroneal	Dorsum of foot, or none
Tibial	Sole of foot

Table 2.5 Sensory loss in the lower limb

3. Examine the sensory system (Table 2.5)

As a minimum check:

a. Light touch and pain sensation over the:
   (i) medial and lateral aspect of the thigh and calf
   (ii) dorsum of the foot, tip of the big toe (L5)
   (iii) lateral border of the foot (S1)
b. Vibration sensation at the medial malleolus
c. Joint position sense at the big toe

4. Test coordination

a. Heel-shin testing
b. Romberg's test
c. Examine the gait (p. 33)

Typical short cases

1. Individual peripheral nerve lesions

Common peroneal (lateral popliteal) nerve

Common short case.

Features
— foot drop: weakness of dorsiflexion and eversion
— usually no sensory loss (Table 2.5)

Causes
— compression of the nerve at the neck of the fibula: e.g. plaster-of-paris cast
— mononeuritis multiplex

Foot drop

Causes   — common peroneal nerve lesion
— sciatic nerve lesion
— peripheral neuropathy
— motor neurone disease
— peroneal muscular atrophy

Sciatic nerve: very rare short case

Features   — complete interruption results in paralysis of all the muscles below the knee — the patient can stand but not up on his toes, and drags the toes of the affected foot as he walks
— absent ankle jerks and plantar reflex
— sensory loss: lateral aspect of the shin, and whole of the foot (except the inner aspect)

Common causes   — trauma: fracture of the pelvis or femur, gunshot wounds of the buttock
— pelvic neoplasm

Tibial nerve: very rare short case

Features   — wasting and weakness of the calf muscles, and muscles of the sole. The foot assumes the position of talipes calcaneovalgus.
— absent ankle jerk and plantar reflex
— anaesthetic sole

Commonest cause   — trauma

Femoral nerve: very rare short case

Features   — wasting and weakness of the knee extensors (quadriceps) and slight weakness of hip flexion. The leg gives way on walking, and the patient is unable to climb stairs.
— absent knee jerk
— sensory loss over the anteromedial surface of the thigh and leg to the medial malleolus

Common causes   — diabetes mellitus
— trauma: fractured pelvis, dislocated hip, or arterial cannulation
— pelvic neoplasm, psoas abscess

2. Spinal root lesions
Very rare short cases. Differ from cervical root lesions in that sensory symptoms are extremely reliable indi-

cators of which root is affected, whilst motor signs are less reliable as most muscles have a nerve supply from two or more roots.

Prolapsed intervertebral discs

Features These can only cause root syndromes (and not spastic paraparesis) as the spinal cord ends at L1. In 95% of cases, the L5 or S1 root is affected. Look specifically for:

1. L5: weakness of the extensor of the big toe.
2. S1: weakness of foot eversion, absent ankle jerk.
3. Straight leg raising limited by pain.

Other causes Very rare, though commoner causes of L2, 3 or 4 root lesions than disc prolapse:
1. Spinal root neurofibroma or meningioma.
2. Metastases.

EXAMINATION OF THE GAIT

Common short case.

Technique Ideally, the patient's feet should be bare, and his legs well exposed. Ask him to walk away from you, turn and then walk back towards you. See if he walks in a straight line; this can be rechecked by asking him to walk along a line on the floor, or heel-to-toe. If he deviates or falls, note to which side. Decide whether the gait conforms to any of the classical types of abnormal gait; if so, look specifically for other features of those conditions.

Typical short cases **1. Cerebellar gait** ('drunken' or 'reeling')
The patient walks with his feet apart and arms outstretched, ready to hold on to any support that is available. He will not fall, but reels consistently to one side (the side of the lesion) if a unilateral lesion is present. The gait is equally severe with the eyes open or closed.

Causes and other features See page 34.

2. Hemiplegic gait ('sticky' gait)
Spastic glutei and quadriceps muscles hold the hip and knee stiff, and spastic plantar flexors keep the foot slightly flexed. Thus the leg describes a semicircle, with the toes scraping the floor (circumduction).

Commonest cause — cerebrovascular accident

3. Paraplegic gait
Spastic gait affecting both legs ('scissors', or 'walking through mud' gait).

Commonest causes
— cerebral palsy
— multiple sclerosis
— cord compression

4. Parkinsonian gait

Difficulty starting ('frozen to the floor') or 'marks time' before beginning to walk. Slow, shuffling gait with small steps ('marche à petit pas'), a slightly stooped posture of the trunk, and arms which are flexed at the elbow and do not swing ('simian posture'). The patient appears to be continuously about to fall forwards. He is unable to stop quickly when pushed forwards (propulsion) or backwards (retropulsion), and finds it easier to walk on uneven ground.

Causes and other features   See page 42.

5. Sensory ataxia (dorsal column loss)

'High-stepping' or stamping gait. The patient walks with a wide base, continuously looking at the ground, raising his feet high in the air and stamping them onto the ground. The gait is greatly accentuated with the eyes closed.

Causes
— tabes dorsalis
— subacute combined degeneration of the cord
— Friedreich's ataxia.

6. Waddling gait ('duck-like')

The feet are planted wide apart, the body is tilted backwards and sways from side to side as each step is taken.

Causes
— congenital dislocation of the hip
— proximal myopathies
— Duchenne muscular dystrophy

7. Foot-slapping gait

In bilateral foot drop, each foot is lifted high in the air (to avoid tripping from catching the toes on the ground), and then slapped back down onto the ground. Unlike in sensory ataxia, the gait is not broad-based, nor is it accentuated with the eyes closed.

Causes
— bilateral peroneal nerve palsies
— peripheral neuropathy (alcoholics)
— progressive muscular atrophy

EXAMINATION OF CEREBELLAR FUNCTION

Common short case.

Technique   Unilateral signs indicate ipsilateral cerebellar disease:
1. Gait ataxia: tendency to deviate towards the affected side on walking.

2. Truncal ataxia: a particular feature of midline cerebellar lesions. Patient may be unable to sit or stand without support, with a tendency to fall backwards. Limb ataxia may be minimal or absent.

3. Limb ataxia:
   a. Observe the outstretched arms: the arm on the affected side tends to hyperpronate, and rise above the other arm. When gentle downwards pressure on the outstretched arm is released, the affected limb flies up out of control.
   b. Finger–nose test: look for incoordination, terminal intention tremor, and past-pointing ('dysmetria').
   c. Heel–shin testing: ask the patient to lift one leg in the air, place the tip of its heel on the knee of the other leg, and then run the heel down the shin. The heel should then be lifted off the shin, and again placed on the knee, and so on (i.e. do not simply ask the patient to rub his heel up and down the other shin). Do not overinterpret minor abnormalities.

4. Rapid alternating movements: ask the patient to rapidly pronate and supinate his wrists ('as if screwing in a light bulb'), play an imaginary piano, tap one hand on the other or his foot on your own hand. Look for any inaccuracy, or fragmentation of movement (dysdiadochokinesia).

5. Test for nystagmus: see page 11.

6. Test for dysarthria: see page 39.

7. Other signs: hypotonia, pendular reflexes (best seen in the knee jerk), enlarged writing.

Common causes — multiple sclerosis: usually also have bilateral pyramidal signs
— anticonvulsant therapy

Rare causes — toxic degeneration: alcohol, carbon monoxide
primary or secondary tumours, non-metastatic manifestation of a malignancy (e.g. bronchogenic carcinoma)
— hereditary ataxia; myxoedema; primary degeneration

EXAMINATION OF INVOLUNTARY MOVEMENTS

TREMOR Common short case.

There are three clinically distinct forms of tremor:

1. Rest tremor

Accentuated when the hands are held outstretched.

Common causes: — physiological tremor: 6–10 cycles per second. More obvious when anxious, in old age, in thyrotoxicosis, and in alcohol intoxication.

— Parkinsonian tremor: rhythmic (3–7 cycles per second), alternating movements of opposing muscle groups (e.g. 'pill rolling'). Usually temporarily suppressed by movement; absent during sleep. Increased by emotional excitement.

— benign essential (familial) tremor: primarily affects the upper limbs, and head (titubation). Increased by emotion and voluntary movement; improved by alcohol. No rigidity or bradykinesia.

Rare causes
— prehepatic coma, uraemia, carbon dioxide retention: 'flapping tremor'
— mercury poisoning ('Hatter's shakes')

2. Intention (action) tremor

Most apparent when, for example, the patient's finger approaches his nose on finger—nose testing.

Causes
— disease of the cerebellum, or cerebellar connections
— Wilson's disease

3. Red nuclear tremor

Most violent type of tremor. Slightest attempt to move a limb is followed by violent, uncontrollable jerking.

Commonest cause
— multiple sclerosis

CHOREA
Rare short case.

Features
The patient appears to fidget continuously. There are sudden, nonrepetitive, involuntary and quasi-purposeful jerks or fragments of movements. These may affect the face (frowning; raising the eyebrows; grimacing, or smiling), tongue or limbs, and are provoked by active movements. Patients often attempt to cover-up an involuntary jerk by performing a voluntary movement (e.g. scratching the cheek).

Causes
— acute rheumatic fever: Sydenham's chorea (St Vitus' dance)
— pregnancy (chorea gravidarum), or use of the contraceptive pill: often have a past history of rheumatic fever
— Huntingdon's chorea: autosomal dominant. Age of onset: 30–45 years. Progressive dementia, with death in 10–15 years
— senile chorea: following a cerebrovascular accident
— rare: thyrotoxicosis, systemic lupus erythematosus, polycythaemia rubra vera

ATHETOSIS	Rare short case.

Features Slower, coarser, more writhing movements of the limbs, face or tongue ('mobile spasm'). Midway between chorea and dystonia.

Causes
— basal ganglia damage: cerebral palsy, kernicterus
— drugs: phenothiazines
— Wilson's disease, Hallervorden-Spatz disease

DYSTONIA	Rare short case.

Features 'Frozen athetosis': prolonged contraction of the trunk or limb muscles, resulting in a distorted posture (e.g. hyperextended neck, plantarflexion of the ankle, oculogyric crisis).

Commonest cause
— drug hypersensitivity or overdosage (phenothiazines, L-dopa, tricyclic antidepressants)
— acute onset dystonia: after a single dose of metoclopramide, or certain phenothiazines (prochlorperazine, fluphenazine)
— tardive dyskinesia: after many years use of certain phenothiazines (e.g. chlorpromazine). Other features include akathisia (fine restless jerkiness of the limbs, inability to sit still), facial spasms, lip smacking, intermittent tongue protrusion and features of Parkinsonism.

Rare causes
— cerebral palsy
— Wilson's disease
— idiopathic torsion dystonia

MYOCLONUS Very rare short case. Brief, repetitive, sudden jerks of a group of muscles, a single muscle or part of a muscle.

Causes
— facial myokymia (e.g. multiple sclerosis)
— epilepsy

HEMIBALLISMUS Very rare short case. Wild flinging movement, usually of an upper limb, following any attempt to move that limb. Invariably unilateral.

Cause
— lesion in the subthalamic nucleus (haemorrhage, infarction)

EXAMINATION OF HIGHER CEREBRAL FUNCTIONS

EVALUATION OF INTELLECTUAL FUNCTION Rare short case. 'Ask this patient some questions'.

Technique

1. Orientation: check if the patient is orientated in time ('what time/day/date/month/year is it?'), and place ('which hospital/ward are you in?').
2. Intellectual function:
   a. Simple calculation: e.g. '100 minus 7' test, simple arithmetic sums.
   b. Immediate recall: ask the patient to repeat a series of numbers (normal: seven numbers).
   c. Short term memory: ask the patient to repeat a lengthy sentence (e.g. Babcock sentence: 'there is one thing a nation must have to be rich and great, and that is a large, secure supply of wood'), or a fictitious name and address, after several minutes.
   d. Long term memory: ask the patient for his date of birth, mother's maiden name, or service number.
   e. General knowledge: e.g. 'name of present/previous Prime Minister/reigning Monarch'.
3. Dysphasia (see p. 40), or dyspraxia: ask the patient to stick out his tongue, make a fist, or flick an imaginary ball.
4. Observe the patient's appearance, and his behaviour and emotional state during the tests.

Typical short case: Dementia

Causes:

1. Often reversible:
   — infections; e.g. neurosyphilis
   — deficiency states: e.g. vitamin B1 or B12, folic acid
   — toxins: drugs, heavy metals
   — metabolic: e.g. hypothyroidism, hypoglycaemia, hypercalcaemia, Cushing's syndrome, liver or renal failure
   — trauma: e.g. subdural haematoma
   — others: hydrocephalus, anoxia, tumours

2. Irreversible:
   — hereditary: e.g. Huntingdon's chorea
   — slow virus infections: e.g. Creutzfeldt-Jakob disease
   — non-metastatic manifestation of malignancy: e.g. bronchial carcinoma
   — others: Alzheimer's or Pick's disease

EXAMINATION OF SPEECH
FUNCTION — SPOKEN
SPEECH

Rare short case. Aim to distinguish defects of articulation (dysarthria), of phonation (dysphonia), or of speech content (dysphasia).

1. Test the power of articulation and phonation
Listen whilst the patient repeats some difficult phrases, e.g.:

East Register Street is opposite West Register Street

Baby hippopotamus
Methodist episcopal
The Middlesex Hospital is in Mortimer Street

Dysarthria

Causes — local lesions in the mouth: e.g. badly fitting false teeth
— bilateral corticospinal tract lesions: e.g. motor neurone disease, vascular lesions of both internal capsules. Other features of pseudobulbar palsy may be present.
— extrapyramidal lesions: e.g. Parkinson's disease: slow, slurred monotonous speech
— disorders of coordination: lesions in the cerebellar vermis or peduncles result in 'scanning' or 'syllabic' speech ('Ba-by hip-po-pot-a-mus'): e.g. multiple sclerosis
— lower motor neurone lesion: bulbar palsy: e.g. progressive bulbar palsy, syringobulbia
— disease of the facial muscles: e.g. myaesthenia gravis (fatiguability may cause increasing slurring), muscular dystrophy

Dysphonia   Normal articulation and speech content, but the patient talks in a whisper.

Causes — laryngitis
— bilateral paralysis of the vocal cord adductors
— hysteria

2. Test for disorders of speech content
a. Test for difficulty in understanding the spoken word (receptive or sensory dysphasia). Having checked the patient can hear, ask him to perform some simple tasks, making sure you do not give any non-verbal clues to your commands: e.g. 'close your eyes', 'touch your nose with your hand', 'pass your watch to me'.
b. Test for difficulty with the expression of speech (expressive or motor dysphasia). Encourage the patient to talk by asking open questions: e.g. 'where do you live?', 'what is your job?', 'what exactly does it entail?'. Listen carefully for defective grammar, jargon, the capacity to finish sentences, any failure in the production of words, incorrect word usage (paraphasia), or the production of new words (neologisms).
c. Test for difficulty in naming objects (nominal dysphasia). Show the patient some common objects and ask him to name them: e.g. a key, 10p coin, the second-hand of a watch. Even if you have already

demonstrated motor aphasia, this test can still be performed by asking the patient to nod when you yourself give the correct name of an object.

Dyphasia	Implies pathology in the left cerebral hemisphere in 93% of right-handed and 40% of left-handed persons: e.g. cerebrovascular accident, tumour.

1. Receptive dysphasia: lesion in the supramarginal gyrus (parietal lobe) and upper part of adjacent temporal lobe (Wernicke's area). May also have an associated visual field defect.
2. Expressive dysphasia: lesion in the inferior frontal gyrus (Broca's area). May also have an associated hemiparesis.
3. Nominal dysphasia: lesion near the angular gyrus.

EXAMINATION OF SPEECH FUNCTION — WRITTEN SPEECH

Unlikely to be asked in a short case. Check the patient's vision before starting. Check for:

1. Visual aphasia (word-blindness): write your commands ('close your eyes', etc) on a piece of paper.
2. Agraphia: ask the patient to write his name and address.

SIGNS OF CEREBRAL HEMISPHERE DAMAGE

Very rare short cases.

Frontal lobe
1. Intellectual impairment, lack of interest, memory defect.
2. Expressive dysphasia (dominant lobe).
3. Loss of smell in one nostril; optic atrophy.
4. Motor deficit: contralateral upper motor neurone signs.
5. Grasp reflexes.

Parietal lobe
1. Receptive dysphasia (dominant) or dyspraxia (non-dominant lobe: e.g. difficulty drawing a clock-face).
2. Inferior quadrantic field defect; attention hemianopia.
3. Cortical sensory loss; sensory inattention.

Occipital lobe
1. Dyslexia or visual agnosia.
2. Homonymous field defects.

Temporal lobe
1. Superior quadrantic field defects.
2. Facial weakness.
3. Hemiparesis (late sign).

NEUROLOGICAL DISEASES

COMMON SHORT CASES   1. PERIPHERAL NEUROPATHY

Features   Motor and sensory signs will vary depending on the disease responsible.

1. Diminished or absent tendon reflexes: if they are all normal, it is most unlikely that the patient has a peripheral neuropathy.
2. Symmetrical, peripheral distribution of muscle wasting and weakness. A predominantly motor neuropathy is seen in porphyria, peroneal muscular atrophy and lead poisoning.
3. Symmetrical sensory loss: all modalities ('glove and stocking'). A predominantly sensory neuropathy is seen in hereditary sensory neuropathy, and some carcinomatous neuropathies (Denny-Brown type).
4. Trophic changes (e.g. ulcers, burns); contractures.
5. Thickened peripheral nerves: amyloidosis, leprosy, Refsum's disease, Dejerine-Sottas disease.

Causes

1. Neural ischaemia: common
— diabetes mellitus
— vasculitis: rheumatoid disease, polyarteritis

2. Genetic: rare
— Dejerine-Sottas disease
— peroneal muscular atrophy
— Friedreich's ataxia
— Refsum's disease (other features, see p. 20)
— hereditary lipoprotein deficiency
— acute intermittent porphyria; variegate porphyria

3. Systemic disease: rare
— carcinoma, reticulosis, paraproteinaemia
— uraemia, liver disease
— acromegaly, myxoedema
— amyloidosis, sacroid

4. Inflammatory or post-infective: rare
— Guillain-Barré syndrome
— leprosy

5. Toxins: rare
— drugs: e.g. isoniazid, nitrofurantoin, vincristine
— heavy metals: e.g. lead

6. Deficiencies: rare
— thiamine: alcoholics
— vitamin B12 or B6

2. PROXIMAL MUSCLE WASTING AND WEAKNESS

Commoner causes   — polymyositis: weakness usually in the pelvic girdle muscles first, then in the shoulder girdle. Rarely affects the external ocular or facial muscles. Tender-

ness of affected muscles (50%). Atrophy is a late sign. Normal reflexes. Look also for a lilac coloured rash on the cheeks and eyelids (heliotrope), and reddened skin over the interphalangeal joints (50%). May have evidence of other systemic connective tissue disease (e.g. scleroderma).
— Cushing's syndrome
— thyrotoxicosis: may be the only overt manifestation
— hypocalcaemia
— carcinomatous neuromyopathy
— diabetic amyotrophy
— hereditary muscular dystrophy: page 46.

3. PARKINSONISM

Features

1. Tremor (p. 36): primarily affects the hands, but may also involve the face and tongue.
2. Rigidity: 'leadpipe' or 'cogwheel'. More obvious when the patient moves the opposite limb (e.g. lifts arm up and down) while tone is being assessed.
3. Bradykinesia: affects mainly the face ('mask facies': infrequent blinking, ocular movements or smiling; persistent glabellar tap reflex), and axial muscles (characteristic posture and gait: p. 34). May also affect speech (quiet, monotonous and slurred), and fine hand movements (e.g. doing up buttons; micrographia).
4. Other features: excessive salivation and dribbling; intellectual impairment (50%); depression; greasy skin.

Causes

— idiopathic (commonest): tremor is usually the first sign. Normal tendon reflexes, and flexor plantar responses.
— drug-induced: e.g. phenothiazines, reserpine. Marked cogwheel rigidity and bradykinesia, with little tremor. Oculogyric crises, and dystonia (p. 37).
— arteriosclerotic: marked rigidity and bradykinesia, with little tremor. Dementia, pseudobulbar palsy, brisk jaw jerk and tendon reflexes, and extensor plantar responses (indicating diffuse cerebral damage). Little or no response to drug treatment.
— postencephalitic: increasingly rare. Oculogyric crises, dystonic postures, and seborrhoeic dermatitis of the face.
— rare causes: manganese exposure; copper or carbon monoxide poisoning; parasagittal meningioma, and meningovascular syphilis

Parkinsonian features may also complicate several rare syndromes:

1. Hepatolenticular degeneration (Wilson's disease)

Autosomal recessive. Age of onset: 10–25 years. Equal sex ratio.

Features Deficiency of caeruloplasmin (the copper-carrying plasma protein) results in copper depositon in the putamen, cornea and liver.
a. Neurological: 'batswing' intention tremor, rigidity, dystonia, and ataxia. Progressive loss of emotional control, and dementia.
b. Eye: Kayser-Fleischer ring. 2 mm diameter zone of golden-brown pigmentation on the posterior surface of the cornea, near the limbus (Descemet's membrane). Rarely: 'sunflower cataract', due to copper deposition in the anterior and posterior lens capsule.
c. Hepatic: cirrhosis.
d. Other features: aminoaciduria, glycosuria.

Prognosis Invariably fatal in 1–6 years until the introduction of D-penicillamine therapy.

2. Shy-Drager syndrome
Parkinsonism with autonomic neuropathy (marked postural hypotension, anhidrosis and impotence).

3. Creutzfeldt-Jakob disease
Parkinsonism with rapidly progressive dementia, spastic weakness of the limbs, and myoclonus.

4. Progressive supranuclear palsy (Steele-Richardson-Olszewski syndrome)
Parkinsonism with marked impairment of eye movements (initially vertical, but later of all voluntary eye movements), and mild dementia.

4. MULTIPLE SCLEROSIS
Areas of demyelination in the CNS, disseminated in time and place.

Commoner features 1. Optic nerve: retrobulbar neuritis (swollen disc, central scotoma), followed by optic atrophy.
2. Brain stem: extraocular nerve lesions (e.g. isolated VIn); internuclear ophthalmoplegia; rotatory nystagmus on lateral gaze; or vertical nystagmus on upward gaze.
3. Cerebellar peduncles: bilateral cerebellar signs (p. 34), almost invariably in association with bilateral pyramidal signs.
4. Spinal cord: dorsal and lateral (pyramidal) tracts; predominantly sensory (paraesthesia; loss of vibration or joint position sense) or predominantly motor signs (pyramidal weakness), or both.

5. Others: Lhermitte's sign (development of electric-like shocks down the body when the patient flexes the head); euphoria, 'scanning' speech; facial myokymia; and urgency or precipitancy of micturition.

RARE SHORT CASES   1. SYRINGOMYELIA

Features   A longitudinal cyst anterior to the central canal in the cervical cord:
1. Cord damage at the root level of the lesion:
   a. Decussating lateral spinothalamic tract fibres: dissociated sensory loss, with painless injuries to the hands, Charcot's joints (e.g. shoulder, wrist).
   b. Anterior horn cells: wasting and weakness of the intrinsic hand muscles, with loss of deep tendon reflexes in the upper limb.
2. Cord damage distant from the lesion: upper motor neurone signs in the lower limbs.
3. Brain stem damage (syringobulbia): Horner's syndrome, loss of pain and temperature in Vb and Vc; bulbar palsy.

2. MOTOR NEURONE DISEASE

Features   The three classical forms reflect degenerative changes in the anterior horn cells, corticospinal tracts and motor nuclei of the lower cervical nerves. Any combination of these three forms may exist. There are *no* sensory changes.

1. Lower motor neurone pattern of weakness, initally of the hands and later of the forearms or shoulder girdles ('progressive muscular atrophy'). Fasciculation is usually prominent; if not, it may be evoked by tapping the muscles.
2. Weakness of the tongue (with wasting and fasciculation), palate and pharyngeal muscles, resulting in dysarthria, dysphagia, nasal regurgitation and a bovine cough ('progressive bulbar palsy').
3. Upper motor neurone pattern of weakness in the legs, spreading to the arms and bulbar muscles ('amyotrophic lateral sclerosis').

Prognosis   Progressive disorder, resulting in death with 2 years in progressive bulbar palsy, and 5 years in progressive muscular atrophy.

3. FRIEDREICH'S ATAXIA
Autosomal recessive. Age of onset 5–15 years.

Features   1. Skeletal: pes cavus, scoliosis.

2. Neurological: progressive degeneration, most marked in the:
   a. Spinocerebellar tracts: cerebellar ataxia, most marked in the legs. Nystagmus (70%), and dysarthria in the later stages.
   b. Dorsal columns of the spinal cord; absent tendon reflexes (ankle disappear before the knee jerks), and sensory impairment (vibration and joint position sense).
   c. Lateral (pyramidal) columns of the cord: upper motor neurone pattern of weakness in the lower limbs, with extensor plantar responses.
3. Other: cardiomyopathy, diabetes mellitus.

Prognosis   Few survive for more than 20 years after the onset of symptoms.

4. PERONEAL MUSCULAR ATROPHY
Charcot-Marie-Tooth disease. Usually autosomal dominant. Age of onset: usually in the 20's.

Features
1. Motor signs predominate: symmetrical wasting and weakness of the peroneal muscles, producing foot drop and pes cavus. Later, there may be atrophy of the calf muscles and distal third of the thigh ('inverted champagne bottle'). Rarely, there is wasting of the distal forearm and small hand muscles.
2. Sensory: vibration sense usually impaired in the legs.
3. Reflexes: usually absent in the legs.
4. Thickened peripheral nerves (25%).

Prognosis   Disease usually arrests spontaneously. Normal life span.

5. SUBACUTE COMBINED DEGENERATION OF THE CORD
Vitamin B12 deficiency: e.g. pernicious anaemia.

Features
1. Neurological:
   a. Degeneration in the dorsal and lateral (pyramidal) columns of the spinal cord: loss of vibration and joint position sense, upper motor neurone pattern of weakness (maximal in the legs), and extensor plantar responses.
   b. Peripheral neuropathy: areflexia; 'glove and stocking' loss of light touch and pain sensation; calves may be tender on deep pressure.
   c. Bilateral optic atrophy (50%); dementia.
2. Other: glossitis, splenomegaly, vitiligo, features of Addison's disease.

Prognosis   With B12 replacement, the neuropathic features improve more completely than the myelopathic.

6. NEUROSYPHILIS

Rarely seen, except as cases of tertiary syphilis with residual signs.

General paresis of the insane   Cortical degeneration

Features
1. Intellectual deterioration: poor memory, lack of concentration, loss of emotional control, delusions, incontinence of urine.
2. Tremor: lips, tongue ('trombone'), hands.
3. Argyll-Robertson pupils.
4. Slurring dysarthria.
5. Pyramidal signs in the legs.

Tabes dorsalis   Degeneration of the dorsal roots, with secondary damage of the dorsal columns.

Features
1. Argyll-Robertson pupils; optic atrophy; ptosis; wrinkled forehead (overactive frontalis muscle).
2. High-stepping gait; ataxia; positive Romberg's sign; loss of vibration and joint position sense in the limbs.
3. Hypotonia; absent tendon reflexes; flexor plantar responses (extensor in taboparesis).
4. Loss of deep pain sensation: nose, sternum, achilles tendon. Trophic foot ulcers; Charcot's arthropathy.

7. MUSCULAR DYSTROPHIES

Dystrophia myotonica   Autosomal dominant. Age of onset: 20–30 years.

Features
1. Neurological
   a. Characteristic expressionless facies and smooth forehead; ptosis, facial weakness. Wasting of the masseters (hollow cheeks), temporalis (hollow temples) and sternomastoids. Cataract (90%). Dementia.
   b. Limbs: wasting and weakness of the shoulder girdle, quadriceps and distal muscles.
   c. Myotonia: delayed voluntary muscular relaxation: e.g. slow relaxation of handshake (long finger flexors).
2. Other: frontal baldness, gynaecomastia, testicular atrophy, diabetes mellitus, cardiomyopathy, abnormal lung function tests (reduced vital capacity), and altered bowel and biliary tree motility.

Prognosis   Slow deterioration. Death within 15–20 years of onset, often from cardiac failure or respiratory infections.

Myotonia congenita   Thomsen's disease. Autosomal dominant. First presents in childhood.

Features   Myotonia: worse in the cold. Improves with procain-amide or quinidine.

Prognosis   Myotonia tends to improve with age. Normal life expectancy.

Duchenne dystrophy   Males, inherited as a sex-linked recessive. Age of onset: 3–10 years.

Features
1. Initial proximal weakness of the limbs, gradually extending peripherally. Rarely affects the hands, face or neck. Absent tendon reflexes, except the ankle jerk. Normal sensation.
2. Hypertrophy of the calves, glutei and deltoids.
3. Waddling gait. Characteristic method of rising from the ground, by 'climbing' up his own legs (weakness of extensors of the spine and knees).
4. Usually of normal intelligence.

Prognosis   Death within 10 years of onset.

Facio-scapulo-humeral dystrophy   Landouzy-Dejerine disease. Usually autosomal dominant. Age of onset: 10–40 years.

Features
1. Weakness begins in the facial muscles; ptosis. Slow progression with increasing weakness and wasting of the neck muscles, sternomastoids, spinati, pectorals, trapezii and deltoids. Pelvic girdle muscles involved late, if at all.
2. Absent biceps and triceps reflexes.
3. May have congenital absence of pectoralis or biceps muscles.
4. Normal sensation, normal intelligence.

Prognosis   Minor disability. Normal life span.

Limb-girdle dystrophy   Usually autosomal recessive. Age of onset: 10–30 years.

Features
1. Slowly progressive wasting and weakness of the shoulder and pelvic girdle muscles. Face never involved. Calves, deltoids and lateral quadriceps may hypertrophy.
2. Impaired proximal tendon reflexes; normal ankle jerks.
3. Normal intelligence.

Prognosis   Often severely disabled in middle life, with death at an earlier age.

3. Cardiovascular system

INTRODUCTION

Almost every candidate is asked to examine some aspect of the cardiovascular system as a short case. Again, you may be asked to perform a complete or only a partial examination of the system: e.g. 'Examine the cardiovascular system' or 'Examine the pulse' or 'the apex beat'. You may even be asked simply to listen to a patient's heart without being allowed to examine the rest of the system, a situation which does not exist in everyday clinical life. You should prepare yourself for this possibility when practising for the short cases.

In the technique for examining the cardiovascular system which follows, I have purposefully tried to include every possible feature which the candidate may face in a short case. In the examination, time would not allow you to look for every feature described, so do not spend very long over, for example, the general inspection, looking at the waveform of the JVP, feeling every arterial pulse, listening for bruits, or palpating for heart sounds and thrills. No mention has been made of percussing the praecordium, as I do not think this is a useful routine part of the physical examination.

EXAMINATION OF THE CARDIOVASCULAR SYSTEM

INSPECTION

Quickly note the following:

Age and general state of the patient

Face

For central cyanosis, anaemia, arcus senilis, xanthalesma, mitral facies; or any features that might suggest a particular syndrome (e.g. Down's syndrome: associated with ventricular septal defect).

Hands

For peripheral cyanosis (low cardiac output), or clubbing, or splinter haemorrhages (p. 133).

Chest wall

For (1) operation scars: e.g. left infra-mammary (closed mitral valvotomy) or central sternal scars (open heart surgery); (2) any asymmetry: e.g. bulge of left chest wall with atrial or ventricular septal defects.

Feet For any obvious ankle swelling, or cyanosis (e.g. in a reversed patent ductus you may see cyanosis, and also clubbing of the feet but not the fingers).

PALPATION 1. ARTERIAL PULSE
Feel the brachial rather than the radial artery. Note:

a. The rate

Bradycardia (rare short case) Rate less than 50 beats minute.

Causes — sinus bradycardia: physical training or drugs e.g. β-blockers, digoxin. Rare causes: myxoedema, jaundice, raised intracranial pressure.
— complete heart block: look for cannon waves in the JVP, and variable intensity of the first heart sound
— 2:1 atrioventricular block, or atrial flutter with 4:1 atrioventricular block (very rare)

b. The rhythm

Atrial fibrillation (rare short case) Pulse irregular in rate and volume. Look for absent *a* waves in the JVP, and variable intensity of the first heart sound.

Common causes — rheumatic valvular disease, especially mitral stenosis
— myocardial ischaemia
— thyrotoxicosis

Rare causes — cardiomyopathy
— atrial septal defect
— constrictive pericarditis
— 'lone' fibrillation

Other causes of an irregular pulse (rare short case) 1. Ventricular extrasystoles: e.g. hypokalaemia, drugs (digoxin).
2. Sinus arrhythmia.
3. Atrial flutter with varying atrioventricular block.
4. Second degree (Wenckebach) heart block.

c. The volume and character (or waveform)
Assess by palpation of the carotid artery.

Typical short cases 1. Large volume pulse (common)
Rapid rate of rise and large volume.

Causes — aortic regurgitation ('water-hammer')
— patent ductus arteriosus
— high output states
— incomplete heart block

2. Small volume pulse (rare)
Implies low cardiac output, e.g. pulmonary hypertension,

pericardial effusion or shock. A small volume pulse with a notch on the upstroke ('anacrotic') and delayed peak ('plateau') is characteristic of severe aortic stenosis.

3. Bisferiens pulse (rare)
Double peak. Feature of combined aortic stenosis and regurgitation.

4. Pulsus alternans (very rare)
In left ventricular failure.

5. Pulsus paradoxus (very rare)
Pericardial effusion, constrictive pericarditis, severe asthmatic attack.

d. The presence and equality of the peripheral pulses
Briefly check at least both radial, brachial, carotid, femoral and posterior tibial arteries. Check for any radiofemoral delay. Briefly listen over both carotid and femoral arteries for bruits.

Unequal pulses
(rare short case)

Causes
— surgical trauma: e.g. previous cardiac catheterisation (via the brachial or femoral artery); Blalock operation
— systemic embolisation: e.g. mitral stenosis
— congenital malformation: e.g. absent radial artery
— aortic dissection
— atherosclerosis

e. Condition of the vessel wall
e.g. thickened wall in longstanding systemic hypertension.

f. Blood pressure
You would not be expected to measure this yourself. Remember to ask the examiner for the value.

2. JUGULAR VENOUS PRESSURE
Remember to have the patient at 45° with his head well supported.

a. Note the height
The distance above the sternal angle (normal: less than 4 cm). Be wary of the grossly elevated JVP: look for movements of the earlobe, or sit the patient up at 90°.

Raised JVP (rare short case)

Causes   — congestive cardiac failure

— fluid overload: e.g. nephrotic syndrome
— hyperdynamic circulation
— rare: superior vena caval obstruction (non-pulsatile); tricuspid stenosis or regurgitation; pericardial effusion

b. Look at the waveform (only very briefly)

Cycle of events: determine their position in the cardiac cycle by simultaneous palpation of the carotid artery.
— *a*-wave: right atrial systole. Absent in atrial fibrillation.
— *c*-wave; tricuspid valve closure (rarely seen).
— *x*-descent (systolic collapse): atrial relaxation and downward displacement of the tricuspid valve towards the right ventricular apex in systole.
— *v*-wave: right atrial filling.
— *y*-descent (diastolic collapse): fall in right atrial pressure when the tricuspid valve opens.
Also:
— *s*-wave: seen in tricuspid regurgitation (not an exaggeration of the normal *v*-wave which occurs later in the cycle).
— *f*-waves: rapid regular pulsations in the supraclavicular fossae, seen in atrial flutter.

Typical short cases (all rare)

1. Exaggerated or giant *a*-waves
Imply that the right atrium is contracting against resistance.

Causes
— tricuspid stenosis
— pulmonary hypertension or stenosis
— large pericardial effusion, constrictive pericarditis

2. 'Cannon' *a*-waves (very rare)
Imply that the right atrium is contracting against a closed tricuspid valve.

Causes
— regular waves: 2:1 atrioventricular block
— irregular waves: complete heart block, extrasystoles

3. Prominent *x*-descent (very rare)
Constrictive pericarditis.

4. Prominent *y*-descent
Constrictive pericarditis
Tricuspid regurgitation.

3. APEX BEAT

a. Determine the position

The lowest and outermost point of definite cardiac pulsation; normally in the 5th intercostal space and within the mid-clavicular line. Define its precise position rather than simply using the term 'apex displaced'.

Typical short cases
1. Impalpable apex beat (common)

Causes
— dextrocardia
— chronic obstructive airways disease
— thick chest wall: e.g. obesity
— congestive cardiac failure
— pericardial effusion (rare)

2. Displaced apex beat (common)

Causes
— cardiac: ventricular enlargement
— non-cardiac: large pleural effusion or pneumothorax, scoliosis, depression of the lower sternum (p. 72)

b. Assess the quality of the cardiac impulse
In a normal heart there is a brief outward movement at the onset of left ventricular ejection. When describing the impulse, avoid physiological descriptions such as 'right ventricular heave'.

Typical short cases
1. Sustained apical thrust (common)
Left ventricular hypertrophy, with or without dilatation.

2. Central thrust or lift in the sternal region (rare), or third or fourth intercostal spaces ('parasternal' heave): right ventricular hypertrophy, with or without dilatation.

3. Abnormal outward systolic pulsation
To the left of the midsternal region (rare): suggests an aneurysm or hypokinetic area of the left ventricular wall.

4. Double apical impulse (rare)
Hypertrophic cardiomyopathy.

c. Feel for any thrills (palpable murmurs or sounds) over the apex and base of the heart
Determine their position in the cardiac cycle by simultaneous palpation of the carotid artery.

Typical short cases
1. Systolic thrill (common)
— at the apex: ventricular septal defect, mitral regurgitation
— at the base: aortic stenosis (to the left) or pulmonary stenosis (to the right)

2. Diastolic thrill (common)
— at the apex: mitral stenosis
— at the base: aortic regurgitation

3. Continuous thrill (rare)
— patent ductus arteriosus (maximum at the left upper sternal border)

4. Palpable heart sounds (rare)
— mitral stenosis: 'tapping' first sound, or palpable opening snap
— pulmonary hypertension: palpable pulmonary sound or ejection click
— ventricular failure: palpable third or fourth sounds
— prosthetic valves

AUSCULTATION

There are a number of basic (but important) points to practise:

— Simultaneously palpate the carotid artery, the best guide to the timing of the auscultatory events.
— Separately listen to each of the auscultatory components, i.e.: Is the first sound normal? Is the second sound normal, and does it split normally? Is there an extra sound in systole, or in diastole? etc.
— Listen over all areas of the heart with both the diaphragm (best for the first and second sounds, any clicks or snaps, and for the murmurs of aortic and mitral regurgitation), and the bell (best for third and fourth sounds, and the murmurs of mitral and tricuspid stenosis).
— Note in your mind accurately what you can hear, and where.
— If appropriate, test the effects of posture (e.g. lying the patient on the left side to accentuate an apical murmur; sitting him upright to listen for a basal murmur), and respiration (right heart noises are louder on inspiration, and left on expiration). You would not be expected to test the effect of exercise or drugs in a short case.
— Finally, you must have made your mind up as to what pathology is present before finishing your auscultatory examination.

1. LISTEN TO THE FIRST HEART SOUND

a. Note its intensity

Typical short cases

1. Loud first heart sound (common)

Common causes

— mitral stenosis
— tachycardia
— prosthetic mitral valve

Rare causes

— atrial septal defect; Wolff-Parkinson-White syndrome (short atrioventricular conduction time).

2. Faint first heart sound (rare)

Common causes   — mitral regurgitation
— myocardial failure

Rare causes   — hypothyroidism
— left bundle branch block
— rheumatic fever (long atrioventricular conduction time)

3. Variable first heart sound (rare)

Causes   — atrial fibrillation or flutter
— complete heart block (and ventricular tachycardia)

b. Note whether it is split to produce two similar high-pitched sounds
This must be distinguished from:

— a fourth heart sound, which is softer
— a presystolic murmur: e.g. mitral stenosis when in sinus rhythm
— an early ejection click, which is higher pitched

Splitting of the first sound (rare)

Causes   — physiological: slight asynchrony in ventricular contraction, e.g. sternal depression
— pathological: mitral stenosis (delayed valve closure), right bundle branch block (delayed right ventricular contraction)

2. LISTEN TO THE SECOND HEART SOUND

a. Note its intensity

Typical short cases   1. Loud second sound (rare)

Causes   — systemic or pulmonary hypertension
— congenital aortic stenosis
— prosthetic aortic valve

2. Soft second sound (rare)

Causes   — calcified or immobile aortic or pulmonary valve

b. Note whether it is split
In some normal people, this may be heard on inspiration over the pulmonary area (aortic component precedes the pulmonary component). A single second sound is heard in older patients, and where either the pulmonary or aortic valve component is inaudible.

Typical short cases

1. Pathological splitting of the second sound (rare)
A split second sound on expiration may be confused with:

— an opening snap: usually later in the cardiac cycle, and associated with a mid-diastolic murmur
— a third heart sound: later, and lower pitched
— a late systolic click (p. 56): higher pitched

Causes

— delay in closure of the pulmonary valve, either due to delayed activation of the right ventricle (e.g. right bundle branch block), or prolonged right ventricular systole (e.g. atrial septal defect, impaired right ventricular function)
— early closure of the aortic valve due to reduced outflow into the aorta: e.g. mitral regurgitation, ventricular septal defect

2. Fixed splitting (rare)
No alteration in the pathological splitting during respiration.

Causes

— atrial septal defect (commonest)
— right ventricular failure

3. Reversed (paradoxical) splitting (rare)
On expiration, the delayed aortic component follows the pulmonary component. On inspiration the aortic component is superimposed on the normal pulmonary component.

Causes

— delay in activation of the left ventricle: e.g. left bundle branch block
— prolongation of left ventricular systole: e.g. severe aortic stenosis, left ventricular outflow tract obstruction, impaired left ventricular function

3. LISTEN FOR ANY EXTRA HEART SOUNDS

a. In diastole

Third heart sound
(rare short case)

Early diastolic triple rhythm. Low-pitched and difficult to hear. Listen with the bell lightly applied to the chest wall. Occurs 0.12–0.16 seconds after the second sound, and is louder with the patient supine, with his legs raised, or after exercise.

Causes

— physiological: healthy people under the age of 40
— pathological: indicates failure from any cause of either the left ventricle (loudest at the apex, on expiration) or right ventricle (loudest at the sternum, on inspiration)

Fourth heart sound (rare)	Presystolic (atrial) triple rhythm.
Causes	— early sign of ventricular disease, either of the left (louder on expiration) or the right (louder on inspiration).
Opening snap (common)	Almost invariably from a stenosed mitral valve (its absence suggests an immobile anterior leaflet due to calcification or stenosis). High-pitched sound, louder on expiration, and best heard with the diaphragm between the apex and the left sternal edge. It is usually followed by a mid-diastolic murmur. Avoid confusing an opening snap with wide splitting of the second heart sound, or an early third sound (p. 55).

b. In systole

Ejection clicks (rare short cases)	Very high-pitched sounds, heard after the first heart sound.
Causes	— aortic click: aortic stenosis (louder on expiration), or regurgitation (if gross, the click may be heard over the peripheral arteries)
	— pulmonary click: pulmonary stenosis (louder on inspiration)
	— similar sounds may occur in dilatation of the aorta or main pulmonary artery
Systolic clicks (rare)	High-pitched sounds, heard in mid or late systole. Characteristic of the mitral valve prolapse syndrome (p. 58).

4. LISTEN FOR ANY MURMURS
For each, note:
— in which part of the cardiac cycle it occurs
— its intensity: grade 1–4
— where it is heard loudest, and where it radiates to
— if appropriate, the effect of respiration or posture

a. In systole

Over the base — aortic area	
Common short cases	— left ventricular outflow tract obstruction
	— aortic cusp sclerosis without stenosis: normal carotid pulse volume, no thrill
	— increased stroke volume ('functional murmur') e.g. aortic regurgitation, anaemia
	— dilated ascending aorta: e.g. systemic hypertension
Rare cases	— coarctation of the aorta
	— vegetations (bacterial endocarditis)
	— acute rheumatic fever

Over the base — pulmonary area

Common short cases	— increased flow across a normal valve: e.g atrial or ventricular septal defect
	— dilated main pulmonary artery: e.g. pulmonary hypertension
Rare cases	— 'Innocent' murmur
	— pulmonary stenosis
At the lower left sternal edge	— ventricular septal defect (common short case)
	— tricuspid regurgitation (rare)
At the apex	— mitral regurgitation (common short case)
	— hypertrophic cardiomyopathy (rare)

b. In diastole

Early diastolic	— aortic regurgitation (common short case)
	— pulmonary regurgitation (rare).

Mid-diastolic (common short case)

Causes	— obstruction: mitral stenosis or aortic regurgitation ('functional' mitral stenosis: Austin Flint murmur). Very rare cases: tricuspid stenosis; mitral valvitis (Carey-Coombs murmur).
	— increased flow: across the mitral valve (e.g. mitral regurgitation; ventricular septal defect; patent ductus arteriosus); or across the tricuspid valve (e.g. atrial septal defect; tricuspid regurgitation)
Late diastolic (presystolic)	— mitral stenosis in sinus rhythm (common short case). Very rare cases: tricuspid stenosis; Carey-Coombs murmur.

c. Continuous murmurs

Common cases	— patent ductus arteriosus
	— aortic stenosis and regurgitation: distinct gap between the systolic and diastolic murmurs
	— ventricular septal defect and aortic regurgitation
Rare cases	— coarctation
	— aorto-pulmonary window
	— ruptured sinus of Valsalva
	— arteriovenous fistula (coronary or pulmonary)
	— venous hum

ABDOMINAL EXAMINATION	If appropriate, palpate for the liver (e.g. pulsatile in tricuspid regurgitation; enlarged in right ventricular failure), spleen (e.g. bacterial endocarditis), or kidneys

(e.g. hypertension: polycystic kidneys, renal artery stenosis), and look for ascites (e.g. constrictive pericarditis).

RESPIRATORY EXAMINATION   If appropriate, listen to the bases of the chest (e.g. pulmonary oedema).

CARDIOVASCULAR DISEASES

COMMON SHORT CASES   1. MITRAL REGURGITATION

Possible features
1. Pulse: quick upstroke ('sharp and abbreviated'); atrial fibrillation occasionally.
2. JVP: normal, unless associated with pulmonary hypertension, cardiac failure or tricuspid regurgitation.
3. Apex: enlarged and hyperkinetic left ventricle. May also feel a systolic thrill or third heart sound.
4. Heart sounds: normal first sound (soft or absent if the valve is calcified or immobile). Second sound normal or widely split (due to shortened left ventricular ejection). May hear a third sound; or one or more midsystolic clicks in mitral valve prolapse syndrome.
5. Murmurs: classically harsh and high-pitched, pansystolic (or late systolic), maximum at the apex and radiating to the left axilla, and louder on expiration. May also hear a short decrescendo diastolic murmur after the third heart sound (increased flow across the valve), or murmurs of other valve lesions (e.g. mitral stenosis).
6. Severity: more severe if there is:
   a. a third heart sound.
   b. an early decrescendo diastolic murmur.
   c. wide splitting of the second sound.
7. Complications: left ventricular or congestive cardiac failure; bacterial endocarditis.

Differential diagnosis
1. Ventricular septal defect: murmur loudest over the left sternal edge; thrill in 90% of cases.
2. Tricuspid regurgitation: prominent v-wave; murmur loudest at the lower left sternal edge and increases on inspiration.
3. Aortic stenosis: slow-rising pulse; low-pitched murmur, of crescendo-decrescendo character, radiating to the carotid arteries.
4. Hypertrophic cardiomyopathy: jerky, ill-sustained pulse of normal volume; double apical impulse; late systolic murmur.

Common causes
— rheumatic mitral valve disease: may also have signs of mitral stenosis or aortic valve disease
— mitral valve prolapse syndrome: associated with

Marfan's and Ehlers-Danlos syndromes, or may occur in normal people. Usually hear one or more midsystolic clicks, sometimes followed by a crescendo-decrescendo late systolic murmur ('honk'). May be complicated by sudden chordal rupture, bacterial endocarditis or sudden death.
— dilatation of valve ring: e.g. left ventricular failure
— papillary muscle dysfunction: e.g. previous inferior myocardial infarction (classically a 'seagull' murmur)

Rare causes   — disease of valve cusps: e.g. bacterial endocarditis, mitral valvotomy, acute rheumatic fever, primum atrial septal defect
— ruptured chordae tendinae or papillary muscles
— Hurler's syndrome, osteogenesis imperfecta, submitral aneurysm
— leaking prosthetic valve

2. MITRAL STENOSIS

Possible features   1. General: mitral facies (more prominent if pulmonary hypertension is present), cold hands, peripheral cyanosis.
2. Pulse: normal character or low amplitude (indicates low cardiac output); atrial fibrillation is common; may have impalpable peripheral pulse or pulses (previous systemic embolisation).
3. JVP: normal, unless associated pulmonary hypertension or tricuspid regurgitation.
4. Apex: usually normal position, unless associated regurgitation or aortic valve disease. May have palpable first heart sound or opening snap, diastolic or presystolic thrill, or left parasternal heave (pulmonary hypertension).
5. Heart sounds: loud 'slapping' first sound (unless the valve is rigid or calcified); normal second sound (unless associated pulmonary hypertension). May hear an opening snap (absent if the valve is rigid or calcified), or rarely a pulmonary ejection click (if associated pulmonary hypertension).
6. Murmurs: classically low-pitched, rumbling, diastolic murmur, loudest at or localised to the apex. Usually mid-diastolic (after the opening snap), with a crescendo presystolic component (if in sinus rhythm). Louder after exercise, and on turning the patient on his left side.
7. Severity: more severe:
   a. The longer the diastolic murmur (unless the cardiac output is low).
   b. The closer the opening snap is to the second heart sound.
8. Complications: atrial fibrillation (common over the

age of 50 years); pulmonary hypertension (features: p. 65); systemic embolisation; angina (due to low cardiac output); venous thrombosis; hoarseness (recurrent laryngeal nerve pressure: Ortner's syndrome); bacterial endocarditis (uncommon in pure stenosis).

Differential diagnosis

1. Aortic regurgitation: Austin Flint murmur. No palpable first heart sound, no opening snap; murmur loudest in midsystole. Third heart sound often present.
2. Secundum atrial septal defect: loud tricuspid valve closure and flow murmur; a fixed split second sound may mimic an opening snap; murmur louder on inspiration.
3. Increased flow across the mitral valve: e.g. mitral regurgitation, patent ductus arteriosus, ventricular septal defect.
4. Left atrial myxoma: diastolic murmur varies with posture.
5. Ball thrombus in the left atrium in mitral valve disease.
6. Cor triatriatum: no murmurs of mitral stenosis.

Commonest cause

— rheumatic valve disease

Rare causes

— congenital: e.g. parachute valve, commissural fusion, Lutembacher's syndrome (mitral stenosis with secundum atrial septal defect)

Combined mitral stenosis and regurgitation

Common, particularly in rheumatic valvular disease. Mitral stenosis is more likely to be the dominant lesion if the pulse volume is small, and the apex is not displaced or hyperkinetic (in the absence of cardiac failure).

3. AORTIC REGURGITATION

Possible features

1. General: may see head bobbing (DeMusset's sign), or capillary pulsation of the nail-beds (Quincke's sign) or retinal vessels.
2. Pulse: rapid upstroke and large amplitude ('water-hammer'). May hear 'pistol-shot' sounds over the brachial or femoral arteries when lightly compressed with the bell; or a to-and-fro bruit over the femoral arteries when lightly compressed with the diaphragm (Duroziez's sign). Wide pulse pressure.
3. JVP: normal venous pressure, unless associated with biventricular failure. May see prominent carotid pulsations (Corrigan's sign).
4. Apex: displaced and hyperkinetic. May also feel a diastolic thrill (along the lower left sternal border),

or systolic thrill (at the base, or over the carotid arteries).

5. Heart sounds: first sound normal or faint (due to premature closure of the mitral valve); second sound normal or absent. May hear third and fourth sounds.

6. Murmurs: high-pitched, blowing, decrescendo diastolic murmur, starting immediately after the aortic component of the second heart sound. Loudest over the lower left sternal edge (listen down all of the left sternal edge with the diaphragm). Louder on leaning the patient forward, and with the breath held in expiration. May also hear an aortic systolic ('functional') murmur, or a mid-diastolic murmur (Austin Flint murmur).

7. Severity: more severe:
   a. The louder or longer the diastolic murmur.
   b. Full, bounding 'water-hammer' pulse.
   c. Low diastolic, and high systolic blood pressure.
   d. Exaggerated arterial pulsations.
   e. Left ventricular hypertrophy or enlargement.

8. Complications: left ventricular or biventricular failure; bacterial endocarditis.

Commonest cause — rheumatic valve disease

Rare causes — congenital: e.g. Marfan's syndrome; bicuspid aortic valve (may be associated with coarctation of the aorta)
— infections: bacterial endocarditis, syphilis
— ankylosing spondylitis; rheumatoid disease; systemic lupus erythematosus; Reiter's syndrome
— leaking prosthetic valve
— trauma; dissecting aneurysm of the ascending aorta

4. AORTIC STENOSIS

Possible features
1. Pulse: slow-rising, small volume pulse, classically with a notch on the upstroke and a delayed peak ('plateau'). May feel a systolic thrill over the carotid arteries. Low blood pressure, with a narrow pulse pressure.

2. JVP: normal, unless associated with biventricular failure.

3. Apex: forceful and sustained. May be displaced (if there is regurgitation or left ventricular failure). May feel a systolic thrill over the base: more obvious with the patient leaning forward with his breath held in expiration.

4. Heart sounds: first sound normal. Normal or loud aortic component of the second sound; soft or absent if the valve is rigid or calcified. May hear a single second sound or paradoxical splitting. May also hear

an ejection click (in a patient under 40 years this suggests the gradient across the valve exceeds 75 mmHg).
5. Murmurs: harsh, 'rasping', low-pitched, crescendo-decrescendo systolic murmur. May be maximum at the upper left or right sternal edge, lower left sternal edge, or at the apex (where it is usually higher pitched and more musical). Radiates to the carotid arteries. May also have murmurs of associated regurgitation or mitral valve disease.
6. Severity: more severe:
   a. The longer the murmur, or the later the peaking in systole.
   b. Palpable or audible fourth sound.
   c. 'Paradoxical' splitting of the second sound.
   d. Left ventricular hypertrophy or failure; murmurs become quieter or may disappear as failure develops.
7. Complications: left ventricular failure; bacterial endocarditis; heart block; sudden death.

Differential diagnosis
1. Mitral regurgitation.
2. Supravalvar or subvalvar left ventricular outflow tract obstruction. Suggestive features are: soft second sound, no ejection click; no valve calcification or post-stenotic dilatation of the ascending aorta on the chest X-ray; characteristic facies in the congenital form of supravalvar stenosis (see below).

Common causes
— calcified bicuspid valve
— rheumatic valve disease
— senile: calcified 'tricuspid' aortic valve

Rare causes
— congenital: unicuspid or bicuspid valve (sometimes associated with coarctation)
— bacterial endocarditis; hyperlipidaemia
— subvalvar aortic stenosis: fixed (e.g. fibrous membrane just below the aortic valve), or variable (e.g. hypertrophic cardiomyopathy)
— supravalvar aortic stenosis: congenital (associated with elfin-like facies, mental retardation and hypercalcaemia), or acquired (e.g. hyperlipidaemia)

Combined aortic stenosis and regurgitation

Common, particularly in rheumatic valvular disease, or in a calcified bicuspid valve. It is the character of the pulse and the blood pressure which are of greatest value in deciding which lesion is dominant. In severe stenosis, there is a small volume pulse, the blood pressure is normal and the pulse pressure narrow. With severe regurgitation, there is a high volume pulse, systolic hypertension and a low diastolic pressure (wide pulse pressure). Though in both conditions the left ventricle may be hypertrophied, it is not usually displaced in aortic stenosis. The loudness of the murmurs are of less value, as a loud systolic flow murmur may be heard in aortic regurgitation when stenosis is absent.

5. VENTRICULAR SEPTAL DEFECT

Features
1. Pulse: prominent upstroke.
2. Auscultation: loud, harsh or blowing, pansystolic murmur (and thrill), loudest at the lower left sternal edge. Split second sound. May also hear a mitral diastolic flow murmur (if the VSD is large).
3. Complications: pulmonary hypertension; reversed shunt (Eisenmenger syndrome: no pansystolic murmur, but systolic murmur from right ventricular outflow obstruction, and signs of pulmonary hypertension); bacterial endocarditis; biventricular failure.
4. Associations: Down's syndrome.

6. 'THIS MAN IS HYPERTENSIVE. EXAMINE HIM'

Technique
1. Look for clues as to the cause of the hypertension: e.g. features to suggest Cushing's syndrome or acromegaly; palpate the abdomen for polycystic kidneys, and listen for a renal arterial bruit; and look for features of coarctation of the aorta (p. 66).
2. Briefly look for complications:
   a. Of the disease:
      (i) Retina: fundoscopy.
      (ii) Cardiovascular system: evidence of left ventricular hypertrophy or failure, or biventricular failure; peripheral vascular disease; previous myocardial infarction (e.g. left ventricular aneurysm).
      (iii) Central nervous system: evidence of previous cerebrovascular accident.
      (iv) Renal impairment or failure.
   b. Of the treatment:
      (i) Bradycardia: e.g. beta-blockers.
      (ii) Extrasystoles: e.g. diuretic-induced hypokalaemia.
      (iii) Postural hypotension: e.g. overenthusiastic treatment.
3. Ask to check present blood pressure, both in the lying and standing positions.

RARE SHORT CASES
1. 'THIS MAN HAS HAD A MYOCARDIAL INFARCTION. EXAMINE HIM'

Technique
1. Look for evidence of possible risk factors:
   a. Cigarette smoking: nicotine-stained fingers, features of chronic obstructive airways disease.

    b. Hypertension: blood pressure reading; complications.

    c. Diabetes mellitus: fundoscopy; urinalysis; complications.

    d. Hyperlipidaemia: arcus senilis; xanthoma or xanthalesma; obesity.

2. Look for complications:

    a. Of the disease:

      (i) Abnormalities of pulse rate or rhythm.

      (ii) Left or right ventricular failure.

      (iii) Papillary muscle dysfunction (mitral regurgitation), or ruptured ventricular septum.

      (iv) Peripheral embolism.

      (v) Left ventricular aneurysm.

      (vi) Pericarditis (p. 68).

    b. Of the treatment:

    e.g. burns on chest wall from previous cardioversion; abdominal wall bruises from subcutaneous heparin injections; scar over femoral artery from previous intra-aortic balloon insertion; sternal scar (previous open heart surgery).

2. 'THIS MAN HAS ANGINA. EXAMINE HIM'

Technique   Look for:

1. Possible risk factors for coronary artery disease: see above.
2. Extracardiac factors which may aggravate any coronary artery disease: e.g. anaemia, thyrotoxicosis.
3. Other causes of angina besides coronary artery disease: e.g. severe aortic valve disease, cardiomyopathy, mitral stenosis, pulmonary hypertension.
4. Complications of the disease (e.g. myocardial infarction) or the therapy (e.g. bradycardia: beta-blocker treatment).

3. CARDIAC FAILURE

Features   1. Left ventricular failure: tachycardia (may feel pulsus alternans); third heart sound; basal crackles, pleural effusion.

2. Right ventricular failure: JVP raised; hepatomegaly; peripheral oedema.

Causes   — disease of heart muscle: ischaemia or infarction. Rarely: myopathy or myocarditis.

    — increased ventricular load:

    a. pressure: e.g. systemic or pulmonary hypertension, aortic or pulmonary stenosis.

    b. volume: e.g. aortic or mitral regurgitation, ventricular septal defect.

c. increased demand (rare): e.g. hyperthyroidism, arterio-venous fistula, anaemia, Paget's disease.
— disorder of rate or rhythm
— combination of the above causes

4. PULMONARY HYPERTENSION

Features
1. General: prominent malar flush, cold extremities, peripheral cyanosis.
2. Pulse: small volume.
3. JVP: prominent a-wave.
4. Apex: left parasternal heave. May also feel the pulmonary component of the second heart sound.
5. Heart sounds: loud pulmonary sound. May also hear a pulmonary ejection click, or right ventricular third or fourth sounds.
6. Murmurs: pulmonary systolic murmur. May also hear an early diastolic murmur (pulmonary regurgitation: Graham-Steell murmur), or systolic murmur of functional tricuspid incompetence.

Causes
— primary pulmonary hypertension
— passive: mitral stenosis, chronic left ventricular failure
— hyperkinetic: congenital heart disease, e.g. ventricular septal defect, patent ductus arteriosus
— vasoconstrictive: chronic obstructive airways disease
— obstructive: emboli (thrombotic, tumour); pulmonary vascular compression and obliteration (e.g. pneumoconiosus)

5. ATRIAL SEPTAL DEFECT

Features
1. Secundum: commoner. Fixed splitting of the second sound. May also hear a pulmonary systolic murmur (due to increased flow). Complicated in middle life by atrial fibrillation, biventricular failure, and pulmonary hypertension. ECG shows right axis deviation and right bundle branch block.
2. Primum: additional mitral pansystolic murmur. Complications arise in adolescence. ECG shows left axis deviation and right bundle branch block.

6. PATENT DUCTUS ARTERIOSUS

Features
1. Pulse: prominent upstroke; prominent pulsation of carotid arteries. Low diastolic pressure.
2. Apex: sustained apical impulse; may also feel a thrill at the upper left sternal edge.
3. Murmurs: harsh continuous murmur ('machinery', 'humming top', 'rolling thunder'), maximum in late systole and loudest at the upper left sternal edge. May

also be heard over the left clavicle, down the left sternal border or at the apex. May also hear an apical diastolic murmur (increased flow across the mitral valve).

4. Complications: pulmonary hypertension (diastolic part of the murmur disappears); Eisenmenger syndrome (cyanosis, and clubbing which may spare the upper body); bacterial endocarditis; biventricular failure.

7. COARCTATION OF THE AORTA

In 98% of cases occurs just distal to the origin of the left subclavian artery.

Features

1. Pulse: disparity in pulsations (diminished femoral pulse, radio-femoral delay) and blood pressures between the arms and the legs (leg systolic pressure normally 20 mmHg greater than in the arm).
2. Apex: sustained apical impulse.
3. Murmurs: continuous, rough murmur, loudest over the spine, or apex of the left lung. May also hear systolic murmurs from frequently associated malformed aortic valve or from dilated collateral vessels (scapular and internal mammary: Susman-Campbell sign — the collaterals may be visible), or diastolic murmurs from malformed aortic valve, or dilated valve ring (systemic hypertension).
4. Associations: polycystic kidney disease, berry aneurysms, Turner's syndrome, neurofibromatosis.

8. TRICUSPID REGURGITATION

Features

1. JVP: prominent s-wave, and may see rapid y-descent.
2. Apex: left parasternal heave; may feel a thrill at the lower left sternal edge.
3. Auscultation: pansystolic murmur at the lower left sternal edge, louder on inspiration (Carvallo's sign). May hear an early diastolic rumble (increased flow across the valve), and a right ventricular third sound.
4. Systolic pulsation of the liver; ascites, peripheral oedema, or a pleural effusion.

Causes

— functional: e.g. due to right ventricular dilatation
— rheumatic valve disease
— others: bacterial endocarditis (main-lining drug addicts); carcinoid syndrome (other features: pulmonary stenosis, flushing, diarrhoea, asthma); trauma; congenital (Ebstein's anomaly)

9. TRICUSPID STENOSIS

Features

1. JVP: elevated; sharp, prominent a-wave, with delayed y-descent.

2. Apex: may feel a diastolic thrill at the lower left sternal edge.
3. Murmurs: presystolic (higher pitched than that of mitral stenosis) and mid-diastolic (loudest between the sternum and the apex); both components are louder on inspiration.

Causes — rheumatic valve disease
— others: carcinoid syndrome, right atrial myxoma, congenital malformation, endomyocardial fibrosis

10. PULMONARY STENOSIS
Very rare short case.

Features 1. Auscultation: normal first and aortic component of the second sound. Ejection click, loudest on inspiration, followed by a harsh crescendo-decrescendo murmur at the upper left sternal edge.
2. Severity: more severe if the following are present:
   a. Left parasternal lift.
   b. Exaggerated a-wave in the JVP.
   c. Longer delay of the pulmonary component after the aortic component of the second sound.
   d. Later peak of the systolic murmur; the murmur may extend beyond the aortic component of the second sound.
   e. Early ejection click: can precede the first sound.
   f. Fourth heart sound.

Causes — acquired: rheumatic valve disease; carcinoid syndrome
— congenital: isolated, part of Fallot's tetralogy, or associated with a ventricular septal defect

11. PULMONARY REGURGITATION

Features Auscultatory signs are very similar to those of aortic regurgitation. The two conditions are distinguished by evidence for aortic regurgitation in the peripheral circulation, or by clinical evidence of pulmonary hypertension.

Causes — pulmonary hypertension
— surgical treatment of pulmonary stenosis; rheumatic valve disease; syphilis; bacterial endocarditis
— congenital: bicuspid valve; associated with a ventricular septal defect .

12. INFECTIVE ENDOCARDITIS

Features Clinical diagnostic tetrad:
1. Heart disease: pre-existing murmur or click; new murmur; cardiac failure; atrial fibrillation. Unusual complication of secundum atrial septal defect, and pure mitral stenosis.

2. Infection: fever, anaemia, sweats, weight loss. Clubbing and splenomegaly may be late signs.
3. Embolism: splinter haemorrhages; mycotic aneurysms; coronary, cerebral, limb, splenic, renal or pulmonary emboli.
4. Immune-complex phenomenon:
   a. Petechial rash: skin and mucous membranes.
   b. Osler's nodes: painful, tender, reddish-brown areas in the pads of the fingers.
   c. Roth's spots: white spots in the retina.
   d. Janeway's lesions: nodular haemorrhagic lesions on the palms or soles.
   e. Haematuria: may be microscopic.
   f. Retinal haemorrhage.
   g. Cerebral vasculitis: psychiatric or neurological syndromes.
   h. Arthralgias.

13. PERICARDITIS AND PERICARDIAL EFFUSION

Very rare short cases.

Features
1. Pericarditis: rub (rough and grating, or superficial and scratchy, or soft and blowing). Listen with the diaphragm pressed firmly against the chest wall, over the base or left sternal edge. The rub is usually tripartite: i.e. in systole, early and late diastole ('triple effect'). Pleural rubs may have a similar quality but are much reduced in intensity when the patient holds his breath.
2. Pericardial effusion: rub disappears; impalpable apex, with increased area of cardiac dullness; soft heart sounds, and may hear a third sound.
3. Cardiac tamponade: JVP raised, with a paradoxical rise on inspiration (Kussmaul's sign). Pulsus paradoxus, and falling arterial pulse pressure. Later stage: tachycardia, with picture of cardiogenic shock.
4. Constrictive pericarditis: JVP raised, with prominent y-descent (and sometimes x-descent). Hepatomegaly, ascites, and less marked ankle oedema. Atrial fibrillation (25%); early diastolic sound (pericardial knock, not third heart sound); impalpable apex.

Causes
— idiopathic
— infection: viral (e.g. coxsackie), bacterial (e.g. tuberculosis), fungal or parasitic
— hypersensitivity: post-infarction or post-cardiotomy; connective tissue disease (e.g. SLE); drug sensitivity (e.g. hydrallazine, procainamide)
— malignancy: e.g. bronchial carcinoma (direct spread or metastases)
— metabolic: e.g. renal failure, hypothyroidism
— trauma: e.g. cardiothoracic surgery
— transudate: e.g. cardiac failure, hypoproteinaemia

14. RHEUMATIC FEVER
Very rare short case.

Features   1. Carditis (75%): aortic or mitral diastolic murmur; cardiac enlargement; pericarditis; heart failure.
2. Arthritis (45%).
3. Chorea (10%).
4. Erythema marginatum (5%).
5. Nodules (15%): 3–4 mm waxy lumps attached to tendon sheaths; over the knuckles, elbows, knees, wrists and back of the head. Last 1–6 weeks.
6. Minor features: arthralgia, fever.

4. Respiratory system

INTRODUCTION Almost every candidate is asked to examine a patient with respiratory signs in the short cases section. This may be quite straightforward, with you being asked to examine the entire respiratory system in a case, for example, of a pleural effusion. An equally common, but far more difficult situation is where you are directed simply to examine part of the system: e.g. 'Examine the chest', or even 'Ausculate the front of this man's chest'.

The cases presented vary from the common clinical disorders (e.g. emphysema; chronic bronchitis; apical fibrosis from healed tuberculosis), to the rare (e.g. bronchiectasis, fibrosing alveolitis), to whatever happens to be on the ward at the time (e.g. resolving pneumonia; pneumonectomy). Some common clinical problems such as asthma are very rarely encountered.

EXAMINATION OF THE RESPIRATORY SYSTEM

INSPECTION

Sputum pot If there is one by the bedside, look in it. This may give an immediate clue to the diagnosis: e.g. mucopurulent sputum would suggest a resolving chest infection; more copious amounts suggests bronchiectasis; the commonest causes of blood-streaked sputum are bronchial carcinoma, pneumonia, pulmonary infarction, bronchiectasis, tuberculosis and mitral stenosis.

Hands Quickly examine the hands for:

1. Nicotine-staining

2. Clubbing

Features
1. Loss of the angle between the nail and nail bed (Lovibond's profile sign).
2. Increased fluctuation of the nail-bed, and an increased ability to 'rock' the nail.
3. Increased curvature of the nail, and an increase in the soft tissues of the end of the finger ('drumstick') are less reliable signs.

Common causes
— bronchial carcinoma
— suppurative lung infection: empyema, lung abscess, bronchiectasis, very extensive pulmonary tuberculosis
— fibrosing alveolitis

Rare causes
— bacterial endocarditis, cyanotic congenital heart disease, atrial myxoma
— inflammatory bowel disease, cirrhosis
— pleural mesothelioma or fibroma; pulmonary secondaries from a primary sarcoma in another organ
— others: familial; idiopathic; hemiplegia (unilateral)

3. Peripheral cyanosis
Compare the patient's nail beds with your own.

Causes
— physiological: cold
— reduced cardiac output: shock, mitral stenosis
— peripheral vascular disease
— causes of central cyanosis: the hands will be warm

4. Briefly feel the pulse
(e.g. 'bounding pulse' in carbon dioxide retention).

Face and neck
1. Look at the conjunctivae for evidence of anaemia

2. Look at the tongue and lips for central cyanosis

Common causes
— chronic obstructive airways disease
— congenital heart disease: VSD, Fallot's
— polycythaemia

Rare causes
— massive pulmonary embolism
— met- or sulph- haemoglobinaemia

3. Note the height and the effect of respiration on the JVP
e.g. right heart failure (look for sacral and ankle oedema, hepatomegaly), superior vena caval (SVC) obstruction.

Chest wall   Remove the patient's clothes from the waist upwards.

1. Note the shape
e.g. scoliosis, kyphosis, thoracoplasty, barrel chest (chronic bronchitis, collapse of the thoracic spine), Harrison's sulcus (severe childhood asthma), pigeon chest, funnel chest (pectus excavatum).

2. Look at the movements
    1. Rate of respiration: normally 14–18 breaths per minute.
    2. Use of the accessory muscles of respiration: sternomastoid, pectoralis, trapezius, and intercostal muscles.
    3. Expansion of the chest wall: note whether the expansion of the two sides is equal. Often more easily seen at a distance from the patient.

Typical short cases   a. Unilateral reduction of chest wall movement

Causes   — pleural effusion
— pneumothorax
— consolidation: pneumonia, tuberculosis, neoplasm or infarction
— collapse, or previous lobectomy or pneumonectomy
— fibrosis: e.g. apical (tuberculosis)

b. Generalised restriction of chest wall movement
Normal expansion is at least 2–3 cm.

Causes   — emphysema
— bilateral pleural effusions
— ankylosing spondylitis

3. Look at the skin
    1. For evidence of previous surgery (thoracotomy, thoracoplasty) or radiotherapy (telangiectasia).
    2. Engorged veins: e.g. SVC obstruction.
    3. Subcutaneous nodules: e.g. metastases.

PALPATION

Determine the position of the mediastinum
1. Upper mediastinum: check whether the trachea is centrally placed within the suprasternal notch, by comparing its distance from the sternomastoid muscles on each side.
2. Lower mediastinum: quickly determine the position of the apex beat.

Typical short case: Mediastinal displacement

Causes   — pleural effusion, pneumothorax ('pushed away')
— fibrosis, collapse, pneumonectomy ('pulled towards')
— tracheal displacement only may occur with upper lobe fibrosis (e.g. healed apical tuberculosis) or collapse, or a large upper mediastinal mass (e.g. retrosternal goitre).

Check the symmetry of movement of the two sides of the chest wall

Test tactile vocal fremitus

Palpate for cervical and axillary lymphadenopathy

PERCUSSION

Percuss by moving down the chest, at the front and back:

Compare the percussion note in comparable areas on the two sides

As a minimum, percuss over each zone and axilla on the two sides.

Map out the limits of lung resonance

1. Apices: remember to tap directly on each clavicle.
2. Bases: on quiet respiration, the lower borders of the lungs lie in the midclavicular line at the sixth rib, the midaxillary line at the eighth, and adjacent to the vertebral column at the tenth rib. The oblique fissure runs from the sixth costal cartilage to one inch lateral to T5 posteriorly; the horizontal runs from the fourth costal cartilage anteriorly and meets the oblique fissure under the fifth rib.
3. Cardiac dullness (rarely necessary): behind the lower left quarter of the sternum.

Typical short cases

1. Increased resonance

Causes

— over large air-filled cavities (e.g. tuberculous, lung abscess), or bullae
— pneumothorax
— emphysema: difficult to appreciate. More reliable signs are the loss of cardiac dullness and the lower limits of lung resonance.

2. Decreased resonance

Causes

— pleural effusion ('stony dull'), or a large fluid-filled cavity
— solid lung tissue: fibrosis, collapse or consolidation (pneumonia, tuberculous, neoplasm, or infarction)
— pleural thickening (e.g. previous tuberculosis)
— raised diaphragm

AUSCULTATION

Listen over each segment of the lung whilst the patient gently breaths in and out through his open mouth. Note the character of the respiratory sounds:

Is the breathing bronchial or vesicular in character?

Bronchial sounds

Produced by the turbulent flow of air through the trachea and major bronchi. The inspiratory sounds becomes inaudible before the end of inspiration (i.e. there is a gap between inspiration and expiration), and the expiratory sound is usually more intense, higher pitched, and more prolonged than the inspiratory sound.

Causes
— over the right apex in normal people
— consolidation; collapse (especially of the upper lobe)
— top of a pleural effusion
— pneumothorax (occasionally)
— large air-filled cavity near the surface of the lung (e.g. lung abscess)

Vesicular sounds
Site of origin remains in dispute (suggestions: turbulent flow in the large bronchi; or laminar non-turbulent airflow in small airways close to the alveoli). The expiratory sound follows that of inspiration without a distinct pause, and is only audible during the earlier part of the expiratory phase. The expiratory sound may be prolonged in asthma and emphysema.

Are the breath sounds diminished or increased in intensity?

Diminished sounds

Causes
— pleural air, fluid or thickening
— pulmonary collapse or fibrosis, lobectomy or pneumonectomy
— bronchopneumonia
— chronic obstructive airways disease

Increased sounds
(usually bronchial in character)

Cause
— consolidation

Are there any added sounds (rales)?
Note their distribution.

Wheezes or rhonchi
Produced by the vibration of the airway walls (like the reed of a wind instrument). May be heard during inspiration and/or expiration.

Causes
1. Generalised:
— smooth muscle contraction: e.g. asthma
— mucous plugging: e.g. chronic bronchitis, emphysema
— pulmonary congestion (occasionally): e.g. left ventricular failure
2. Localised:
— local bronchial obstruction: e.g. carcinoma, inflammation, lymph node, foreign body

Crackles or crepitations
Produced by the explosive re-opening of collapsed airways ('opening snaps').

Causes	1. Finer crackles: — lung fibrosis: e.g. fibrosing alveolitis (usually late in inspiration, and disappear when the patient leans forward), or previous apical tuberculosis — pulmonary oedema (usually early in inspiration) — early or resolving stages of pneumonia — lung collapse (occasionally) 2. Coarser crackles: — chronic bronchitis (usually early inspiratory and late expiratory) — bronchiectasis
Pleural rub or friction sounds	Dry pleurisy.
Note the character and intensity of the vocal resonance	Ask the patient to say '99', whilst you listen over each lung zone and the axillae with your stethoscope.
Typical short cases	1. Diminished vocal resonance and tactile vocal fremitus
Causes	— pleural effusion (may have a bleating character just above the fluid level: 'aegophony') — pneumothorax — collapse, pneumonectomy, fibrosis (may be increased)
	2. Increased vocal resonance (bronchophony) and tactile vocal fremitus
Causes	— consolidation ('whispering pectoriloquy') — fibrosis (occasionally) — collapse (occasionally: especially the upper lobe)

RESPIRATORY DISEASES

COMMON SHORT CASES	1. PLEURAL EFFUSION
Features	See Table 4.1.
Common causes	1. Transudate: — cardiac failure 2. Exudates: — inflammation: pneumonia, tuberculosis — neoplasm: pleural metastases (lung, breast, ovary) — pulmonary infarction
Rare causes	1. Transudate: — hypoproteinaemia (nephrotic syndrome, cirrhosis) 2. Exudates: — inflammation: lung or subphrenic abscess, acute pancreatitis — neoplasm: primary pleural tumours — collagen disorders: rheumatoid disease, SLE

— trauma: following a lobectomy or pneumonectomy; contusion; oesophageal rupture
— complicating ascites: Meig's syndrome (ovarian fibroma)

	Consolidation	Collapse or removal	Fibrosis	Pleural effusion	Pneumothorax
Mediastinal shift	None	Towards	Towards	Away	Away
Tactile vocal, fremitus or vocal resonance	Increased	Usually diminished bronchophony (upper lobe)	Diminished or bronchophony	Diminished (aegophony)	Diminished
Percussion note	Dull	Dull	Dull	'Stony' dull	Tympanic
Breath sounds	Bronchial	Absent or bronchial (upper lobe)	Diminished or bronchial	Diminished*	Diminished
Added sounds	Fine inspiratory crackles during early stages and resolution	None	Fine late inspiratory crackles	None	none or click†

* May hear bronchial breathing at the upper level of the dullness
† In a left-sided pneumothorax, a click synchronous with cardiac systole may be heard

Table 4.1 Classical physical signs in chest diseases

2. CHRONIC OBSTRUCTIVE AIRWAYS DISEASE

Features   Two patterns can be recognised clinically, though many patients display some features of both:

Chronic bronchitis ('blue bloaters')

1. Heavier build. Cyanotic. Plethoric. Loud breathing.
2. Barrel chested.
3. Quiet vesicular breath sounds, often with early inspiratory and late expiratory coarse crackles, and expiratory wheezes.
4. Complications:
   a. Cor pulmonale.
   b. Respiratory failure: peripheral vasodilatation (warm hands, bounding pulse, engorged retinal veins), and varying degrees of agitated confusion. Late signs: flapping tremor of outstretched hands, papilloedema, coma.
   c. Pneumonia.

Emphysema ('pink puffers')

1. Thin. Not cyanosed.
2. Breathless. Pursing of the lips during expiration. Use of the accessory muscles of respiration.
3. Hyperinflation of the chest:
   a. Increased resonance on percussion (difficult to appreciate).

b. Diminished cardiac and hepatic dullness. Low posterior basal resonance.
c. Indrawing of the lower intercostal spaces and the supraclavicular fossae on inspiration.
d. Shortening of the cricosternal distance to less than the normal 2–3 fingers breadth.
e. JVP rises on expiration.
4. Quite vesicular breath sounds, with prolonged expiratory phase, often with scattered expiratory wheezes.

RARE SHORT CASES

1. FIBROSING ALVEOLITIS

Features (Table 4.1)

1. Clubbing (60%). Central cyanosis.
2. Classically: fine persistent basal end-inspiratory crackles which disappear on bending far forward.
3. Complications: cor pulmonale, respiratory failure.

Causes of diffuse lung fibrosis

— cryptogenic (fibrosing alveolitis); connective tissue disorders (e.g. rheumatoid disease, SLE, scleroderma)
— inhaled inorganic dusts: asbestosis, silicosis
— inhaled organic dusts: extrinsic allergic alveolitis (e.g. Farmer's lung)
— ingested toxins: busulphan, nitrofurantoin, cyclophosphamide, paraquat
— infections: miliary tuberculosis or histoplasmosis
— miscellaneous: sarcoidosis, haemosisiderosis, radiation damage

Causes of localised lung fibrosis

— healed tuberculosis: apices
— bronchiectasis, or previous severe infections
— ankylosing spondylitis: upper lobes

2. BRONCHIECTASIS

Features

1. Copious mucopurulent sputum (± haemoptysis).
2. Central cyanosis, clubbing, halitosis.
3. Reduced chest wall movements.
4. Dull percussion note, diminished tactile vocal fremitus and vocal resonance.
5. Reduced breath sounds, with coarse crackles (usually over the bases: see below). Bronchial breathing may be heard over a consolidated area.
6. Complications: fibrosis, cor pulmonale, lung or brain abscess, amyloidosis.

Common causes

— following childhood respiratory infections: e.g. whooping cough, measles
— previous tuberculosis: often only affects the right middle lobe, or the anterior segment of the upper and lower lobes

— cystic fibrosis: autosomal recessive. Equal sex incidence. Onset in early childhood. Other features: pancreatic malabsorption (weight loss, steatorrhoea), cirrhosis

— proximal bronchial obstruction: e.g. foreign body, bronchial carcinoma

Rare causes

— congenital: Kartaganer's syndrome (autosomal recessive: situs inversus, absent frontal sinuses, immobile spermatozoa), or Williams-Campbell syndrome (congenital absence of cartilage distal to the first division of the peripheral bronchi)

— congenital or acquired hypogammaglobulinaemia

— bronchopulmonary aspergillosis

3. PNEUMONIA

Lobar pneumonia (with the classical signs of consolidation: Table 4.1) is unlikely to be seen as a short case. Very rarely, the candidate is asked to examine a case of resolving pneumonia (e.g. in a chronic bronchitic, or postoperative patient), or of atypical pneumonia (Mycoplasma pneumonia. Other very rare features of mycoplasma infection: hepatitis, splenomegaly, generalised lymphadenopathy, pericarditis, cerebellar ataxia).

4. PNEUMOTHORAX

Features

1. Table 4.1
2. Complications: tension pneumothorax (cyanosis, gross mediastinal displacement, evidence of circulatory collapse); mediastinal or subcutaneous (surgical) emphysema.

Common causes

— spontaneous: tall young men

— ruptured emphysematous bullae

— trauma: e.g. fractured rib, open wound

Rare causes

— tuberculosis: often also have a small pleural effusion

— asthma

— cavitating pneumonia: *Klebsiella*, *Staphylococcus*

— bronchial carcinoma

— occupational lung disease

— artificial ventilation

— miscellaneous: neurofibromatosis, pleural endometrioma

5. TUBERCULOSIS

Possible features

1. Old apical tuberculosis, with resultant fibrosis (Table 4.1), or cavity formation.
2. Bronchiectasis, especially of the right middle lobe.
3. Previous therapy: thoracoplasty, plombage.

6. SARCOIDOSIS

Possible features

1. Respiratory: signs are notably absent, unless pulmonary fibrosis (Table 4.1) supervenes.
2. Skin:
   a. acute: erythema nodosum.
   b. chronic: lupus pernio, scar infiltration.
3. Eyes: uveitis, choroiditis; or band keratopathy (hypercalcaemia).
4. Enlarged salivary glands.
5. Hepatosplenomegaly, slight peripheral lymphadenopathy.
6. Bone sarcoid: swollen, red finger ends.
7. CNS: isolated peripheral or cranial (especially VIIn) palsies; diabetes insipidus.

7. BRONCHIAL CARCINOMA

Possible features

1. Respiratory: clubbing, hypertrophic pulmonary osteoarthropathy, collapse, consolidation or an effusion (Table 4.1).
2. Local spread:
   a. SVC obstruction: cyanosis and oedema of the face, neck and arms; distended non-pulsatile external jugular veins; enlarged and tortuous anastomotic veins on the anterior chest wall; bilateral exophthalmos and papilloedema (very rare). Other causes: enlarged thyroid or thymus gland, large pericardial effusion.
   b. Horner's syndrome.
   c. Pancoast's tumour.
   d. Hoarseness; dysphagia.
   e. Atrial fibrillation, pericarditis or pericardial effusion.
3. Metastases: cervical and axillary lymph nodes, brain, liver, bone, skin.
4. CNS: dementia, cerebellar degeneration, peripheral neuropathy, proximal myopathy, polymyositis, Eaton-Lambert syndrome.
5. Endocrine: gynaecomastia; ectopic hormone production (ACTH, ADH).
6. Skin: dermatomyositis, acanthosis nigricans, migratory thrombophlebitis.
7. Anaemia, weight loss.
8. Treatment: pneumonectomy, lobectomy, radiotherapy.

5. Abdomen

Almost every candidate will be asked to examine a patient's abdomen as a short case. By far the likeliest abnormality to be found will be an enlarged liver, spleen or kidney. Cases of pancreatic and intestinal pathology (e.g. steatorrhoea; inflammatory bowel disease) are rarely, if ever, seen. In the genito-urinary system, besides enlargement of one or both of the kidneys, the only case you are likely to see is of a patient with chronic renal failure.

EXAMINATION OF THE ABDOMEN

INSPECTION

General Briefly look for the following:

1. General: loss of weight; pigmentation (e.g. uraemia, primary biliary cirrhosis; not haemochromatosis); stigmata of chronic liver disease (Table 5.1).
2. Eyes: jaundice; anaemia; Kayser-Fleischer rings; xanthalesmata.
3. Mouth:
   a. Tongue: degree of hydration; colour (e.g. pale and atrophic in iron deficiency; 'raw beef' in B12 deficiency; magenta in riboflavin deficiency).
   b. Foeter: e.g. uraemia ('fishy'), hepatic failure ('mousy').
   c. Angular cheilitis: e.g. iron deficiency, dentures.
   d. Peri-oral pigmentation: Peutz-Jegher syndrome (p. 98).
   e. Inspection of the teeth, gums, palate, fauces and pharynx is not required in this situation.
4. Hands: clubbing (e.g. cirrhosis; inflammatory bowel disease); koilonychia (iron deficiency); leuconychia (hypoalbuminaemia); brown line near the end of the nails (chronic renal failure).

Abdomen The patient must be lying flat on his back, quietly breathing through his open mouth, with no more than one pillow under his head, and his arms by his side. The whole of the abdomen and lower chest should be exposed, down to just above the top of the pubic region.

Stigmata	Other causes
Spider naevi (on the area of skin drained by the superior vena cava)	Pregnancy, contraceptive pill
Palmar erythema	Rheumatoid disease, SLE Pregnancy Chronic leukaemia, bronchial carcinoma Thyrotoxicosis
Scattered telangiectasia on the face	Progressive systemic sclerosis Hereditary haemorrhagic telangiectasia (Osler-Rendu-Weber syndrome: may also have hepatosplenomegaly) Systemic lupus erythematosus Rosacea Outdoor occupation
Testicular atrophy; sparse axillary and pubic hair	Klinefelter's syndrome
Gynaecomastia	Drugs: e.g. spironolactone, digoxin, stilboestrol Endocrine: e.g. adrenal tumours, acromegaly, thyrotoxicosis Klinefelter's syndrome Bronchial carcinoma Physiological: e.g. puberty
Central cyanosis	Page 71
Clubbing	Page 70
Leuconychia	Nephrotic syndrome Hypothyroidism
Purpura, bruising	Page 99
Dupuytren's contracture	Peyronie's disease Familial/Idiopathic (may also have knuckle pads over the PIP joints of the fingers: Garrod's knuckle pads) Retroperitoneal fibrosis
Bilateral parotid swelling	Page 131
Flap (asterixis)	Uraemia

Table 5.1 Stigmata of chronic liver disease

1. Look for swelling: either general (fluid, fat, flatus, faeces or fetus), or local (e.g. hepatomegaly; abdominal mass; incisional hernia).
2. Look for epigastric pulsation: e.g. aortic pulsation in a thin patient; aortic aneursym; tumour overlying the aorta; hepatic venous pulsation (tricuspid regurgitation).
3. Look at the skin for:

a. Distended surface veins:
Determine the direction of blood flow.

Causes   — portal hypertension: flow away from the umbilicus. Rarely, distended veins radiating from the umbilicus (Caput Medusae) may be seen.
— inferior vena caval obstruction: flow is upward from the groin
— superior vena caval obstruction: dilated veins on the chest and upper abdomen. Flow is usually downward.

b. Operations

Scars; colostomy (usually on the left) or ileostomy (usually on the right); shunts (e.g. LeVeen: peritoneojugular).

c. Visible peristalsis

e.g. small bowel obstruction.

PALPATION   Before starting, ask the patient whether he has any abdominal discomfort, and to indicate where it is. Use the flat surface of your fingers, not their tips (except when palpating for specific organs). Ensure your hand is warm before touching the patient.

1. Gently palpate the whole of the abdomen (i.e. all nine zones), avoiding any painful area until last. Note any local or general rigidity, or marked tenderness.
2. Repeat the process, with firmer, deeper palpation, feeling for any abnormal masses. If present, note their position, size, consistency, shape, motility and percussion note.
3. Palpate for internal organs:

Liver   a. Before palpation, percuss the liver area so not to miss a grossly enlarged liver, or situs inversus. The upper border usually reaches to the fifth intercostal space, so begin higher up and percuss downwards in the midclavicular line. To define the lower edge, percuss upwards from the resonant bowel areas (looking for any evidence of a previous liver biopsy at the same time). In a non-emphysematous patient, the normal liver does not extend beyond one centimetre below the costal margin on deep inspiration.

b. On palpation, note the following:

— Is the liver enlarged? Note by how much (express in centimetres or finger-breadths below the costal margin), and whether the enlargement is general or localised (e.g. tumour, Riedel's lobe).
— The character of the edge and surface: e.g. soft, smooth and tender (heart failure, acute hepatitis); firm and finely nodular (cirrhosis); hard and coarsely irregular (metastases, macronodular cirrhosis).
— Is the liver pulsatile? e.g. tricuspid regurgitation.

Typical short cases   1. Hepatomegaly (common)

Common causes   — cirrhosis (page 85): alcoholic (or alcoholic steatosis), haemochromatosis
— right heart failure
— lymphoma; myeloproliferative disease (e.g. polycythaemia rubra vera)

Rare causes
— primary biliary cirrhosis
— carcinoma: metastases, hepatoma
— infections: e.g. glandular fever, hydatid cyst, amoebic abscess, infectious hepatitis
— constrictive pericarditis; tricuspid regurgitation; hepatic vein thrombosis
— polycystic disease of the liver (and kidney): autosomal dominant inheritance in the adult form
— miscellaneous: collagen disease (e.g. Felty's syndrome; Still's disease); amyloidosis; sarcoidosis; glycogen storage diseases: fatty infiltration (cachexia)
— Riedel's lobe: tongue-like extension of the right lobe of the liver. Commoner in women. May be mistaken for a liver tumour or an enlarged right kidney.

2. Hepatosplenomegaly (common)

Causes
— myeloproliferative disease: e.g. myelofibrosis, chronic myeloid leukaemia
— portal hypertension
— chronic heart failure
— lymphoma
— infection: e.g. glandular fever
— amyloidosis
— anaemia: e.g. pernicious anaemia

Spleen
Do not start palpating too near the costal margin, otherwise an enlarged spleen will be missed. A slightly enlarged spleen can best be felt if the patient half rolls over onto his right side.

Splenomegaly (common short case)

Features
a. Dull percussion note.
b. The spleen enlarges diagonally downwards, across the abdomen, in line with the ninth rib.
c. The edge is sharp and distinct, and a notch can often be felt though not invariably.
d. You cannot palpate above the swelling.
e. Moves downwards on inspiration.

Causes
a. Gross enlargement
— common: chronic myeloid leukaemia, myelofibrosis
— rare: malaria, kala-azar
b. Moderate enlargement: lymphoma, chronic lymphocytic leukaemia, portal hypertension.
c. Slight enlargement: any of the above; infections (e.g. glandular fever, infectious hepatitis, brucellosis, bacterial endocarditis); collagen disease (e.g. Felty's syndrome); amyloidosis; polycythaemia rubra vera.

Kidneys   Palpate bimanually. The lower pole of the right kidney can usually be felt in thin normal people.

Enlarged kidney(s) (common short case)

Features   a. Overlying percussion note is resonant.
b. Rounded edge, with no notch.
c. Can feel above the upper border.
d. Moves slightly downwards on inspiration.

Causes   a. Bilateral enlargement:
— polycystic kidney disease: autosomal dominant inheritance in adults. Other features: berry aneurysms, polycystic disease of the liver.
— bilateral hydronephrosis
— amyloidosis
b. Unilateral enlargement (rare short case):
— cysts
— hydronephrosis
— renal carcinoma
— hypertrophy of a single functioning kidney

Gall bladder   Impalpable, unless distended. Situated just to the lateral side of the right rectus muscle, adjacent to the ninth costal cartilage (Murphy's sign: tenderness on palpation on inspiration).

Intestines   Palpate for abnormal masses, especially in the epigastrium (e.g. gastric carcinoma; pancreatic cyst), and suprapubically (e.g. uterine fibroids). The descending colon is often palpable in the left iliac fossae of normal people.

4. Examine for **ascites**: look for shifting dullness, or try to elicit a fluid thrill (requires a larger volume of fluid). In the presence of gross ascites, the edge of an enlarged organ (e.g. the liver) may be felt by 'dipping' (ballottement).

Common causes   — intra-abdominal neoplasms
— hepatic cirrhosis with portal hypertension

Rare causes   — cardiac: right heart failure; constrictive pericarditis
— hypoproteinaemia: nephrotic syndrome
— peritoneal dialysis
— peritonitis: bacterial, tuberculous

5. Ask the examiner if he wants you to examine the hernial rings and external genitalia.
6. Ask whether there was any abnormality on rectal examination.

7. If appropriate, feel for cervical lymphadenopathy (e.g. intra-abdominal carcinoma: Troisier's sign), or generalised lymphadenopathy (e.g. hepatospleno-megaly).

AUSCULTATION

1. Bowel sounds; succussion splash in pyloric obstruction.
2. Liver: systolic bruit (hepatoma; alcoholic liver disease); friction rub (hepatoma; liver biopsy).
3. Kidneys: renal artery stenosis.
4. Umbilicus: venous hum over collaterals in portal hypertension.

ABDOMINAL DISORDERS

COMMON SHORT CASE   CIRRHOSIS OF THE LIVER

Features   The liver is palpable in most cirrhotics. A very large liver suggests haemochromatosis or alcoholic cirrhosis (or steatosis), whereas a small shrunken liver is indicative of cryptogenic cirrhosis. Look for evidence of a previous liver biopsy. Other features are determined by the following complications:

Hepatocellular failure

1. Jaundice.
2. Spider naevi (more than five); white spots on the arms and buttocks; palmar erythema; scattered telangiectasia on the face ('paper-money' sign); loss of forearm, axillary, chest and pubic hair; testicular atrophy; gynaecomastia.
3. Central cyanosis (intrapulmonary shunts); clubbing.
4. Leuconychia (may also see horizontal white bands across the distal part of the finger nails) and peripheral oedema (hypoalbuminaemia); bruising (decreased synthesis of clotting factors).
5. Hepatic foetor ('mousy').
6. Flapping tremor (asterixis): flexion–extension at the metacarpophalangeal and wrist joints. Ask the patient to extend his arms, separate the fingers, and forcibly, dorsiflex the wrist. This posture may have to be maintained for 15 seconds or more before the flap is seen.
7. Other signs of encephalopathy (intellectual impairment, cerebellar features).
8. Marked muscle wasting.

Portal hypertension

1. Ascites (may also have abdominal herniae).
2. Splenomegaly.
3. Spontaneous portocaval anastomoses:
   a. Anterior: umbilical vein connects the left branch of the portal vein to the abdominal wall veins,

which are dilated (may also have a thrill and venous hum). Blood flow is away from the umbilicus.

   b. Inferior: inferior mesenteric vein connects the splenic vein to the rectal and anal venous network.

   c. Superior: right gastric vein connects the portal vein to the azygous vein through the gastric and oesophageal venous network.

   d. Posterior: posterior gastric vein connects the splenic vein to the inferior vena cava through the gastric venous network, left suprarenal vein and left renal vein.

4. Haemorrhage from the oesophageal or gastric varices; or from a peptic ulcer (which are more common than in the general population).

Other causes of portal hypertension

All rare. Cirrhosis accounts for 90% of cases in adults.

1. Suprahepatic obstruction:
— in the main hepatic veins: Budd-Chiari syndrome (e.g. neoplasm; polycythaemia rubra vera; contraceptive pill; ulcerative colitis)
— in the centrilobular venules: veno-occlusive disease (e.g. ingestion of alkaloids: ragwort plant)

2. Intrahepatic obstruction:
— cirrhosis
— non-cirrhotic: congenital hepatic fibrosis, hepatic schistosomiasis (*S. Mansoni*)

3. Infrahepatic obstruction:
— congenital malformation of the portal vein
— portal vein compression: e.g. pancreatic carcinoma
— invasion of the lumen of the portal vein: e.g. hepatoma
— portal vein thrombosis: e.g. umbilical sepsis

Other complications of cirrhosis

— infection
— hepatoma: heralded by a sudden clinical deterioration: e.g. appearance of ascites; fever; rapidly enlarging liver. Listen for a systolic bruit over the liver.
— pancreatitis

Types of cirrhosis

1. Cryptogenic: commonest.

2. Alcoholic: usually micronodular. Other possible features: florid spider naevi, and bruising (due to repeated falls); bilateral, painless parotid enlargement; fever; Dupuytren's contractures; nutritional deficiencies (e.g. red tongue; wet beri-beri; Korsakoff's psychosis; Wernicke's encephalopathy; peripheral neuropathy); and a systolic bruit over the liver.

3. Chronic active hepatitis: often macronodular.
   a. 'Lupoid': usually young females. Other features:

moon-shaped facies, acne and abdominal striae (looks like Cushing's syndrome); polyarthropathy. May be associated with thyroiditis, ulcerative colitis, renal tubular acidosis, fibrosing alveolitis, diabetes mellitus and haemolytic anaemia.

b. Hepatitis B antigen positive: usually males. Commonly develop a hepatoma.

c. Drug-induced: e.g. methyldopa, oxyphenisatin, isoniazid, aspirin.

4. Haemochromatosis: males, over the age of 30 years. Originally thought to be autosomal dominant mode of inheritance. Portal hypertension and hepatocellular failure are not common. Other features: slate-grey skin pigmentation; diabetes mellitus (50%); polyarthropathy (chondrocalcinosis: 55%); testicular failure and impotence (68%); cardiac failure or arrhythmias (4%).

5. Wilson's disease: page 42.

6. Primary biliary cirrhosis. Middle-aged females. Other features: multiple scratch marks (early pruritis: may result in lichenification); xanthelasmata and xanthomas (especially over sites of trauma or pressure: e.g. venepuncture); skin pigmentation (spares old scars; may also be present in the nails), and rarely hypertrophic osteoarthropathy. May be associated with progressive systemic sclerosis, Sjögren's syndrome, and thyroiditis.

7. Others: secondary biliary cirrhosis; alpha-1-antitrypsin deficiency; glycogen storage diseases; galactosaemia; cystic fibrosis.

RARE SHORT CASES 1. 'THIS MAN IS JAUNDICED. EXAMINE HIM'

Technique Look for the following possible features:

1. Eyes: depth and type (see below) of jaundice; anaemia; Kayser-Fleischer rings (Wilson's disease); xanthalesmata (primary biliary cirrhosis).

2. Face, chest, upper limbs:
   a. Stigmata of chronic liver disease.
   b. Needle punctures (drug addicts); tattoos.
   c. Purpura, bruising, scratch marks.

3. Neck: palpate for lymphadenopathy (e.g. intra-abdominal neoplasm; lymphoma).

4. Abdomen:
   a. Skin: operation scars (e.g. cholecystectomy); collateral circulation (portal hypertension).
   b. Hepatomegaly: e.g. cirrhosis, metastases.
   c. Splenomegaly: e.g. portal hypertension, hereditary spherocytosis.
   d. Distended gall bladder: implies extrahepatic biliary obstruction (Courvoisier's law).

e. Ascites.

f. Inguinal lymphadenopathy.

g. Ask the examiner for the result of the rectal examination: e.g. pale faeces; rectal carcinoma; metastasis in the pouch of Douglas.

5. Legs: ankle swelling, scratch marks, ulcers (e.g. sickle cell disease).

6. Nervous system: flap, encephalopathy.

Causes

1. Prehepatic or unconjugated jaundice: light lemon yellow colour.

— haemolysis: e.g. sickle cell disease, hereditary spherocytosis

— Gilbert's syndrome (affects 2–5% of the population): defective hepatic uptake and conjugation of bilirubin, shortened red cell survival. Probably autosomal dominant inheritance.

— drugs: e.g. novobiocin

2. Hepatocellular jaundice: orange yellow colour.

— cirrhosis; chronic active hepatitis

— alcoholic liver disease

— hepatitis: viral; glandular fever; Weil's disease (leptospirosis)

— drug hepatotoxicity: dose dependent (e.g. paracetamol) or independent (e.g. monoamine oxidase inhibitors, halothane)

— congenital (very rare): Crigler-Najjar (absent conjugating enzyme), and Dubin-Johnson syndrome (defect in excretion of bilirubin: greenish-black liver on biopsy)

3. Cholestatic jaundice: greenish-yellow colour.

a. Intrahepatic:

— primary biliary cirrhosis

— drugs: e.g. phenothiazines, oral contraceptives

b. Extrahepatic: biliary obstruction: e.g. gallstones; pancreatic or biliary tree carcinoma; stricture or compression of the common bile duct.

2. 'THIS PATIENT IS ANAEMIC. EXAMINE HIM'

The aim of your examination is to note (a) the features of anaemia, (b) the pathophysiological consequences, and (c) any features which suggest the cause.

Technique

Look for the following possible features:

1. General: racial origin (e.g. Negro: sickle cell disease; Mediterranean: thalassaemia); pallor of the skin and conjunctivae; fever; blue eyes and white hair (pernicious anaemia).

2. Face: jaundice (haemolysis); angular stomatitis, and pale atrophic tongue (iron deficiency); 'raw beef' tongue (B12 deficiency); stigmata of chronic liver

disease, hereditary haemorrhagic telangiectasia, or hypothyroidism.
3. Hands: koilonychia (iron deficiency); chronic arthropathy.
4. Cardiovascular system: haemodynamic consequences (e.g. heart failure, tachycardia, systolic flow murmur).
5. Abdomen: hepatomegaly, splenomegaly, tumour masses, operation scars (e.g. partial gastrectomy); ask for details of the rectal examination (e.g. melaena).
6. Legs: ulcers (e.g. sickle cell disease).
7. Nervous system. For completeness, ask the examiner if he wants you to examine for evidence of subacute combined degeneration of the spinal cord (B12 deficiency) or fundal haemorrhages (severe anaemia).
8. Lymphadenopathy; breasts (carcinoma).

Causes
1. Acute or chronic blood loss.
2. Impaired red cell formation:
— genetic disorder of haemoglobin synthesis: e.g. thalassaemia
— deficiency of substances essential for erythropoiesis: e.g. iron, B12, folate
— anaemia of chronic disorders: e.g. infection, inflammation, malignancy, renal or hepatic disease
— aplastic anaemia; bone marrow infiltration (e.g. leukaemia, myeloma, myelofibrosis)
— endocrine disorders: e.g. hypothyroidism, hypopituitarism
3. Haemolytic anaemia.

3. 'THIS PATIENT IS URAEMIC. EXAMINE HIM.'

The aim of your examination is to note (a) any features which suggest the cause, (b) any complications, and (c) evidence of treatment.

Technique
Look for the following possible features:
1. Skin: dryness; colour ('dirty yellow pallor' pigmentation in chronic cases); scratch marks; purpura.
2. Mouth: breath ('fishy').
3. Hands: leuconychia; brown line near the end of the finger nails; flap.
4. Cardiovascular system: pericarditis; features of hypertension and its possible complications; evidence of fluid overload (sacral, ankle oedema; raised JVP), or depletion (postural hypotension; cold peripheries); haemodialysis access (shunt, fistula).
5. Abdomen: enlarged kidneys (e.g. polycystic disease, bilateral hydronephrosis); evidence of previous peritoneal dialysis, or renal transplantation.

6. Nervous system: mental state; peripheral neuropathy.

Causes   — glomerulonephritis (40%)
          — pyelonephritis (11%)
          — polycystic disease of the kidneys (9%)
          — diabetic nephropathy (9%)
          — hypertensive nephrosclerosis (7%)

6. Skin

INTRODUCTION   Patients with skin diseases are commonly used as short cases, though they differ from those involving other systems in two main respects. Firstly, they are usually 'spot diagnoses'. Secondly, the cases provoke many more questions from the examiner, for example, on differential diagnoses, other features, and occasionally on treatment.

Although common in clinical practice, skin infections and infestations are very rare short cases. You should, however, be able to recognise these conditions as well as those mentioned in this chapter. If not familiar with these diseases by direct experience, consult an atlas of dermatology (see bibliography).

EXAMINATION OF A PATIENT WITH A SKIN DISORDER

Technique   1. Identify the form of the individual skin lesions: Table 6.1.
   2. Define its distribution, e.g.
      a. Extensor surfaces: psoriasis, dermatitis herpetiformis.
      b. Flexor surfaces: lichen planus, erythema multiforme.

Lesion	Examples
Macule: circumscribed alteration in the colour of the skin, with no elevation	Purpura (does not blanch with pressure) Erythema (eg drug reaction) Pigmentation
Papule: circumscribed palpable elevation, less than 1 cm diameter	Lichen planus
Nodule: palpable mass greater than 1 cm in diameter	Neurofibromatosis
Wheal: area of oedema	Urticaria
Vesicles, bullae: accumulations of fluid within or below the skin	Herpes simplex Pemphigus, pemphigoid
Pustule: visible accumulation of pus	Acne vulgaris Pustular psoriasis
Scales: accumulation of excess keratin	Ichthyosis ('lizard' skin) Psoriasis Tinea infection
Ulcer: full-thickness circumscribed loss of skin	Varicose ulcer

Table 6.1 Forms of individual skin lesions

    c. Unilateral segmental eruption: herpes zoster.

    d. Linear lesion: Koebner phenomenon (psoriasis, lichen planus, molluscum contagiosum, viral warts, sarcoidosis).

3. Having made the diagnosis or a list of differential diagnoses, look specifically for other features of each disorder, e.g.:

Nail involvement	— psoriasis — lichen planus (10%) — vitiligo — Reiter's disease
Joint involvement	— psoriasis — rheumatoid disease (nodules) — gout (tophi) — inflammatory bowel disease (pyoderma gangrenosum)
Eye or eyelid involvement	— erythema multiforme — rosacea — pemphigus vulgaris — xanthomas (arcus senilis, xanthalesma)
Alopecia	— systemic lupus erythematosus — lichen planus
Mouth lesions	— lichen planus — pemphigus vulgaris — erythema multiforme

SKIN DISEASES

COMMON SHORT CASES

Common short cases

1. PSORIASIS

Affects 2–3% of the UK population. Familial tendency. Characterised by well-defined areas of thickened red skin, with loosely applied, silvery scales.

Features

Three main types:

1. Chronic nummular (discoid): commonest form. Discs or plaques of affected skin, classically on the extensor aspects of the limbs, the sacral area and the scalp.

2. Acute guttate (L. drop): small, sharply circumscribed lesions scattered evenly over the body. Usually occurs in adolescence, often following a streptococcal sore throat. In contrast, the lesions in **pityriasis rosea** are oval, with centripetal scaling, and are concentrated on the trunk with their long axes parallel to the ribs.

3. Flexural psoriasis: axillae, groins, submammary folds and umbilicus. In these moist situations, the lesions do not become scaly. Their sharply demarcated edges

help differentiate it from seborrhoeic dermatitis or moniliasis.

Other features, complications

1. Koebner phenomenon.
2. Nail involvement: 30% have typical pinpoint pits ('thimble-like') in some or all of their nails. Less common features are transverse ridges, thickening under the nail, and onycholysis.
3. Pustular psoriasis:
   a. Chronic: firm sterile pustules on the palms or soles (similar appearance to pompholyx); or
   b. Acute and generalised.
4. Generalised exfoliative psoriasis (erythroderma): page 102.
5. Psoriatic arthropathy: page 111.

2. DERMATITIS (or eczema: *Gk*. bubbling, boiling)

Features

Areas of erythema with vesiculation, exudation, crusting and excoriation. Chronic eczema is thicker, dryer and cracked. The distribution depends on the type of dermatitis.

1. Atopic: in the older child and adult, the skin is drier, thickened (lichenification: Besnier's prurigo) and often pigmented, and affects the face, popliteal and cubital fossae, wrists and ankles.
2. Allergic or irritant contact dermatitis: e.g. rubber gloves (hands), nickel (under the buttons and studs of jeans; car-lobes; wrists); cosmetics or antibiotic drops (eyelids).
3. Seborrhoeic: greasy, yellowish, scaly eruption of the scalp, eyebrows, nasolabial folds, ears, centre of the chest and back, submammary areas, axillae and groins.
4. Varicose (gravitational): scaly eruption of the lower limbs associated with venous stasis and pigmentation.
5. Nummular (discoid): coin-shaped eruptions, symmetrically distributed on the limbs.
6. Pompholyx: soles, palms, and sides and front of the fingers.
7. Photosensitive: light-exposed areas; e.g. reaction to drugs (phenothiazines, sulphonamides, nalidixic acid), pellagra.

RARE SHORT CASES

1. LICHEN PLANUS

Features

1. Itchy eruption of highly characteristic lesions: purplish, flat-topped, shiny papules (1–2 mm diameter, polygonal in outline and often umbilicated). Some larger papules have white lines passing through them (Wickham's striae). The papules may be arranged in rings of 1–2 cm diameter (annular type: not to be confused with **granuloma annulare** in

which annular purplish papules are present on the
dorsa of the hands).
2. Distribution:
    a. Chronic: Flexor aspects of the wrist and forearms,
       trunk and lower limbs (where the papules tend to
       be larger).
    b. Acute, generalised type.
3. Koebner phenomenon.
4. Mouth lesions (25%): delicate, white striae, or profuse
   white dots (resembles candidiasis, but immobile) on
   the buccal mucosa. Usually asymptomatic. May
   occur in the absence of the skin lesions.
5. Nail involvement (10%): longitudinal ridging and
   splitting.
6. Lichen planus-like eruptions can be drug-induced:
   e.g. gold, methyldopa.

2. ACNE VULGARIS
Age of onset: adolescence. Equal sex incidence.

Features   1. Comedones, papules and pustules. Also cysts in
                  severe cases.
               2. Distribution: face, back of neck, chest and back
                  (areas rich in sebaceous glands).
               3. Unusual causes:
                   a. Drugs: steroids, contraceptive pill, phenobarbitone.
                   b. Cushing's syndrome.
                   c. Industrial acne: e.g. chlorinated hydrocarbons.
                   d. Stein-Leventhal syndrome: obese, hirsute and
                      infertile women with polycystic ovaries.

3. ROSACEA
Age of onset: 30–50 years. Commoner in women.

Features   1. Papules and pustules, and rarely cysts; no come-
                  dones. Underlying erythema, with telangiectasia.
               2. Distribution: flush areas of the forehead, nose,
                  cheeks, and chin. Rarely, also on the neck, upper
                  chest and arms.
               3. Less common features: rhinophyma; eye involve-
                  ment (conjunctivitis, keratitis); eyelid involvement
                  (blepharitis, lymphoedema).

4. ERYTHEMA NODOSUM

Features   1. Sudden onset of painful, tender, erythematous,
                  saucer-like nodules (3–4 cm diameter) on both shins,
                  and very occasionally on the thighs or extensor
                  aspects of the arms. When it fades, it looks like a
                  normal bruise.
               2. May have associated ankle oedema and arthralgia,
                  and fever.

Common causes — streptococcal infection: e.g. sore throat, tonsilitis
— drugs: contraceptive pill, sulphonamides
— sarcoidosis.

Rare causes — other bacterial infections: tuberculosis, leprosy (especially when under treatment with dapsone), brucellosis
— inflammatory bowel disease
— lymphoma, leukaemia, Behçet's syndrome, fungal infections (e.g. histoplasmosis)

5. ERYTHEMA MULTIFORME
Young adults and children: commoner in women.

Features

1. Acute onset of a variety of lesions: pink macules or papules; annular red lesions, sometimes with a purple centre ('target lesion'), or in severe cases a vesicle or bulla in the centre.
2. Distribution: face, flexor aspects of the forearms, hands, and feet.
3. Mucous membrane involvement: buccal mucosa may be shed, leaving a raw red surface. Similar changes may occur on the vulva, and there may be urethritis.
4. Eye involvement: conjunctivitis.
5. Stevens-Johnson syndrome: all of the above, with fever and arthralgia.

Common causes — virus infection: herpes simplex
— drugs: barbiturates, sulphonamides

Rare causes — bacterial infection: streptococcus, mycoplasma pneumonia
— SLE
— pregnancy
— leukaemia, ulcerative colitis, X-ray therapy

Other conditions with ocular, oral and genital involvement

1. Reiter's disease.
2. Behçets syndrome.
3. Pemphigus vulgaris.
4. Toxic epidermal necrolysis (Lyell's syndrome).

6. VESICLES, BLISTERS OR BULLAE

Causes

Physical

1. Friction, insect bites, burns, cold..
2. Light sensitivity: erythema and blistering in areas exposed to light, particularly the face and dorsum of the hands.
   a. Drugs: tetracyclines, sulphonamides, phenothiazines, thiazides, nalidixic acid.
   b. Plants: e.g. parsnips.

        c. Porphyria cutanea tarda or variegata.
        d. Pellagra.

Chemical 1. Contact dermatitis, pompholyx.
2. Fixed drug eruptions: e.g. salicylates, barbiturates.

Bullous diseases in adults 1. Dermatitis herpetiformis
Subepidermal blisters. Age of onset: 20–40 years.
Features 1. Clusters of very itchy blisters on an erythematous
background.
2. Bilateral, symmetrical distribution: extensor surfaces
of the elbows and knees, and buttocks.
3. Association with glutein-sensitive enteropathy.

2. Pemphigus vulgaris
Intra-epidermal blisters. Age of onset: 40–60 years.
Features 1. Very painful bullae usually first appear in the mouth.
May also have genital blisters (especially on the
vulvae).
2. Flaccid blisters, on normal looking skin, heal without
scarring. Little or no irritation. Nikolsky's sign (may
produce the bullae by gentle rubbing of normal
skin).

3. Pemphigoid
Subepidermal blisters. Age of onset: 60–80 years.
Features 1. Tense blisters, which occur on areas of erythema.
Usually first appear on the leg or arm.
2. No mucous membrane involvement.

Infections 1. Bullous impetigo.
2. Herpes simplex or zoster: may be generalised in an
immunosuppressed patient.

Others Erythema multiforme, lichen planus, herpes gastationis,
severe vasculitis (haemorrhagic blisters, with ulcers)

7. SUBCUTANEOUS NODULES (also p. 103).

Causes 1. Rheumatoid nodules
Particularly over the dorsal apsect of the elbow.

2. Gouty tophi
On the ear cartilages, and close to affected joints.

3. Subcutaneous calcinosis
Progressive systemic sclerosis (or in the CREST
syndrome). Other features: page 109.

4. Neurofibromatosis (Von Recklinghausen's disease)
Autosomal dominant.

Features   a. Skin: pedunculated nodules, axillary freckling (Crowe's sign), and café au lait macules.
b. Nervous system: peripheral neurofibromata; intracranial (e.g. VIIIn glioma and intraspinal tumours).
c. Other: phaeochromocytoma; medullary carcinoma of the thyroid; uterine fibromas.

5. Xanthomas
Three types:
a. Yellowish sheets on the eyelids (xanthelasma: p. 17), palms or neck; usually also have arcus senilis. Commonest in type IIB lipoproteinaemia: associated with coronary artery disease, hypertension, and diabetes mellitus.
b. Large nodules (tuberous) on the extensor surfaces or over tendons. Feature of type IIA lipoproteinaemia: primary, or secondary to prolonged cholestasis, hypothyroidism, nephrotic syndrome.
c. Crops of small red or yellow papules (eruptive). Feature of type IV lipoproteinaemia: primary, or secondary to diabetes mellitus, obesity.

6. Lipomas
Multiple in Dercum's disease.

7. Acute rheumatic fever (p. 69)

8. AREA OF DECREASED PIGMENTATION

Causes   **1. Circumscribed**

Congenital

Common: Vitiligo   Affects 1% of the population of the UK: family history in 35%. Usually begins before the age of 20.

Features   — bilateral, symmetrical areas of depigmentation, occasionally with hyperpigmented borders
— affects the backs of the hands, forearm, face, axillae and genitalia
— associated with thyroid disease, diabetes mellitus, Addison's disease, pernicious anaemia, and alopecia areata

Rare   — tuberose sclerosis: 'ash leaf' depigmented macules (90%), usually on the lower trunk and buttocks. Other features: adenoma sebaceum of the face, periungual fibromata, irregular coarsened skin over the sacrum (shagreen patch), epilepsy and mental deficiency.

— piebaldism: triangular white fore-lock of hair and normal pigmentation of the hands and feet.

Acquired

Common
May follow virtually any inflammatory disorder: e.g. SLE; herpes zoster; burns; pityriasis alba (cheeks and upper arms of adolescents)

Rare
— pityriasis versicolor: superficial skin infection with *Mallasezia furfur*. White or light brown, slightly scaly 'rain-drop' lesions on the chest, trunk and neck.
— tuberculoid leprosy: lesions have an anaesthetic centre
— morphoea (localised scleroderma); plaques of hardened skin, sometimes with a violet-coloured halo
— chemical depigmentation: e.g. hydroquinine, cloroquine

2. Generalised

Congenital (very rare)
— albinism: autosomal recessive. Milk-white skin, white hair, blue irides, red pupils and characteristic bright red fundi. May also have nystagmus and photophobia.
— phenylketonuria

Acquired (rare)
— hypopituitarism; previous arsenic therapy ('raindrop' appearance)

9. AREA OF INCREASED PIGMENTATION

Causes
1. Circumscribed

Congenital
1. Café au lait patches: may find up to 5 in otherwise normal people. Feature of neurofibromatosis, Albright's syndrome (polyostotic fibrous dysplasia: with multiple bone lesions and sexual precocity in females).
2. Lentigo type:
   a. Peutz-Jegher syndrome: autosomal dominant. Lentigines around the mouth, on the buccal mucosa and dorsa of the fingers. Associated with benign hamartomata in the small bowel.
   b. Leopard syndrome (very rare): L = lentigines (very numerous, scattered all over the body); E = ECG abnormalities; O = ocular defects; P = pulmonary stenosis; A = abnormalities of genitalia; R = retardation of growth; D = deafness.
3. Chloasma type: pregnancy, drugs (contraceptive pill,

phenytoin). Irregular macular hyperpigmentation confined to the forehead, upper lip and cheek.

Acquired 1. Following many skin diseases or trauma (common): e.g. herpes zoster, eczema, lichen planus, fixed drug eruptions (e.g. phenolphthalein, sulphonamides), or heat (e.g. erythema ab igne).
2. Acanthosis nigricans (very rare): adenocarcinoma (e.g. stomach), Cushing's syndrome, obesity, acromegaly, or drugs (e.g. nicotinic acid). Dark, velvety thickening of the skin in the axillae and groins.
3. Malignant melanoma.

2. Generalised

Endocrine 1. Addison's disease: also prominent brown or blue macules on the gums and buccal mucosa.
2. Nelson's syndrome; ACTH and MSH secreting tumours.
3. Thyrotoxicosis.
4. Acromegaly.

Metabolic 1. Liver disease (e.g. prolonged cholestasis); haemochromatosis ('bronze diabetes').
2. Chronic renal failure.
3. Porphyria cutanea tarda: facial bullae (heal with scarring) and hypertrichosis; Nikolsky's sign.
4. Pellagra.

Drugs Chlorpromazine (slate-grey hyperpigmentation, confined to exposed areas), busulphan, gold and silver (argyria: slate-grey).

Scleroderma

Malignancy, malnutrition

10. PURPURA, ECCHYMOSES

Causes **1. Vessel (capillary) disorders**

Congenital (very rare) Ehlers-Danlos syndrome. Other features: hyperextensible joints, poor wound healing, easily stretchable skin, blue sclerae and aortic dissection.

Acquired 1. Increased permeability (very rare): e.g. scurvy: perifollicular petechiae, particularly on the legs; larger ecchymoses, swelling of the gums, loss of teeth.
2. Increased fragility (common): e.g. senile purpura; Cushing's syndrome or steroid treatment; diabetes mellitus; uraemia.

3. Chronic venous stasis (common): gravitational (varicose) eczema.
4. Vasculitis (rare): e.g. Schönlein-Henoch purpura: children or young adults. Palpable purpura most profuse on the feet and legs, and occasionally the upper limbs. Other features: arthropathy, renal involvement (from microscopic haematura to acute glomerulonephritis), gastrointestinal involvement (abdominal pain, melaena).

2. Blood disorders (very rare short case)

Platelets
1. Thrombocytopenia: e.g. idiopathic; bone marrow disease (e.g. leukaemia) or suppression (e.g. cytotoxics); systemic disease (e.g. SLE); splenomegaly.
2. Qualitative platelet defect: e.g. hereditary thrombasthenia.

Dysproteinaemias   e.g. cryoglobulinaemia.

Coagulation disorders   e.g. anticoagulant treatment (e.g. subcutaneous heparin injections); hypoprothrombinaemia (e.g. liver disease, bowel sterilisation)

Diffuse intravascular coagulation   e.g. meningococcal septicaemia.

11. URTICARIA
Eruption of itchy, circumscribed, oedematous swellings which last for a few hours.

Types
1. Allergic (acute) urticaria: drugs (e.g. penicillin, aspirin), foods (e.g. tartrazine).
2. Toxic urticaria: nettles, insect bites.
3. Urticaria induced by pressure (dermographism); light; cold (may be due to circulating cryoglobulins or cold agglutinins); heat or emotion (cholinergic).
4. Hereditary angioedema: C1 esterase inhibitor deficiency.
5. Chronic (idiopathic) urticaria.
6. Initial manifestation of systemic vasculitis: e.g., SLE, Schönlein-Henoch purpura, polyarteritis nodosa. Urticaria is usually more persistent and tender than the other types, lasting for several days.

12. DISORDERS OF THE NAILS
1. Infection: candida (chronic paronychia; onycholysis); tinea (onycholysis); bacterial endocarditis (splinter haemorrhages; other causes: p. 133).
2. Associated skin disease: psoriasis (pitting, onycholysis); lichen planus (longitudinal ridges); alopecia areata and vitiligo (pittong, shedding).

3. Associated systemic disease: any severe illness (transverse furrows: 'Beau's line'); iron deficiency anaemia (koilonychia); thyrotoxicosis or hypothyroidism (onycholysis); Reiter's disease (subungual separation).
4. Trauma: nervous habit of flicking one nail with another (multiple transverse ridges or white bands: 'ladder deformity').
5. Ischaemia: Raynaud's phenomenon, progressive systemic sclerosis (excessive longitudinal ridging, and thinning of the nails).
6. Colour changes:
   a. Brown nails: chronic renal disease.
   b. White nails: hypoalbuminaemia, hypothyroidism.
   c. Yellow nail syndrome: increased transverse curvature, gross thickening and yellow discolouration. May be associated with bronchiectases, idiopathic pleural effusions, lymphatic oedema, and myxoedema.
7. Median canaliform dystrophy: 'inverted fir tree' appearance. Idiopathic.
8. Drugs: cloxacillin, cephaloridine (onycholysis).

13. DISORDERS OF HAIR

Alopecia

Types
1. Diffuse loss on the frontal regions and vertex: 'normal' male-pattern baldness
2. General thinning or loss of hair:

Causes
— endocrine: post-menopausal, myxoedema, hypopituitarism, hypoadrenalism
— drugs: cytotoxics (e.g. cyclophosphamide), anticoagulants, contraceptive pill, sodium valproate
— iron deficiency anaemia
— acute hairfall: following parturition or an acute illness

3. Loss of hair in well-defined patches.

Causes
— alopecia areata: 'exclamation mark' hairs. Often associated with vitiligo, thyroid disease, pernicious anaemia, and Down's syndrome.
— ringworm
— trauma

4. Scarring alopecia

Causes
— trauma: burns, scalds
— SLE
— sepsis: boils, ringworm (kerion)
— lichen planus; herpes zoster
— very rare: lupus vulgaris, syphilis

Hirsutism

Common causes
— constitutional: racial, familial
— Cushing's syndrome
— drugs: phenytoin, steroids, minoxidil, streptomycin, diazoxide, androgens

Rare causes
— tumours: adrenal, ovarian (e.g. arrhenoblastoma)
— Stein-Leventhal syndrome (p. 94)
— congenital adrenal hyperplasia
— porphyria cutanea tarda (p. 123)

Features which suggest virilisation
— temporal baldness
— deepening of the voice
— breast atrophy
— masculine habitus
— clitoral hypertrophy

14. ERYTHRODERMA ('homme rouge'; generalised exfoliative dermatitis)

The whole of the patient's skin is red and oedematous, and sheds a large amount of scale. May be complicated by heart failure (due to the large increase in skin blood flow), hypothermia, malabsorption and gynaecomastia.

Causes
— complication of an underlying skin disease (70% of cases): eczema, psoriasis
— lymphoma, leukaemia
— drugs: penicillin, sulphonamides, streptomycin, gold, phenylbutazone

7. Joints

INTRODUCTION Patients with rheumatic diseases are only occasionally used as short cases. You are unlikely to be asked simply to examine one joint, although obviously you must be prepared for this possibility. A commoner approach is for the examiner to ask you to look at a patient's hands or feet. Once a 'spot diagnosis' has been made, be prepared to demonstrate or list the other features of the disorder, or important differential diagnoses.

EXAMINATION OF THE JOINTS Always compare the corresponding joints on the two sides of the body.

1. INSPECTION AND PALPATION
Look for:

Swelling May be bony (e.g. Heberden's nodes, Charcot's joints), or due to soft tissue swelling or fluid (e.g. inflammatory arthropathy).

Deformity
1. Malalignment of articulating bones (e.g. ulnar deviation of the fingers in rheumatoid disease; kyphosis or scoliosis of the spine).
2. Alteration in the relationship of the two articulating surfaces (e.g. subluxation, dislocation).

Changes in the overlying skin:
1. Redness or increased warmth: acute inflammatory reaction: e.g. septic arthritis, gout.
2. Subcutaneous nodules: rheumatoid nodules, gouty tophi. Rare causes: systemic lupus erythematosus, polyarteritis nodosa, rheumatic fever, multicentric reticulohistiocytosis.
3. Scars: e.g. synovectomy (rheumatoid disease), arthrodesis.
4. Rash: see below.
5. Oedema: sign of acute inflammation (e.g. early rheumatoid arthritis).

Muscle wasting Intrinsic muscles of the hands (e.g. rheumatoid disease), quadriceps (painful knee joint).

Tenderness around the joint For example, synovial inflammation, inflamed Heberden's nodes, bony spurs.

2. TEST THE RANGE OF MOVEMENTS (Tables 7.1–7.3)

Before beginning, always ask the patient whether the joint is painful.

a. Test both passive and active movements: estimate the range of movement (you would not be expected to use a goniometer or protractor).

b. Note whether there is any discomfort on movement.

c. Test the stability of the joint.

d. Feel for any crepitus.

The range of movement may be increased in hypermobility syndromes (e.g. Marfan's or Ehlers-Danlos syndrome, Osteogenesis imperfecta).

Cervical spine	Rotation	60°	'Look behind you to the left (right)'
	Flexion	45°	'Look down'
	Extension	45°	'Look up'
	Lateral bending	45°	'Put your right ear on your right shoulder'
Thoracic spine	Look for kyphosis or scoliosis		
	Rotation of the head and shoulders with the patient sitting		
	Chest expansion: measure with a tape measure. Normal lower limit = 5 cm.		
Lumbar spine	Flexion		'Touch your toes'
	Extension		
	Lateral bending		'Slide your right (left) hand down your leg'
Sacroiliac joints	Test for irritability:		
	a. with the patient supine, press the iliac crests towards each other ('springing the pelvis').		
	b. downward pressure on the sacrum with the patient prone.		

Table 7.1 Examination of individual joints: spine

Shoulder	Abduction	180°
	Adduction	50° 'Carry your arm across the front of the chest'
	External rotation	60°
	Internal rotation	90° 'Scratch your back'
	Flexion	90°
	Extension	65°
Elbow	Flexion	150°
	Hyperextension	0°
	Pronation	80°
	Supination	90°
Wrist	Extension (dorsiflexion)	70°
	Flexion (palmarflexion)	70°
	Radial deviation	20°
	Ulnar deviation	30°
Fingers	Flexion at the metacarpophalangeal and interphalangeal joints	
Thumb	Extension	
	Flexion	
	Opposition	
	Adduction	

Table 7.2 Examination of individual joints: upper limb

Hip	Trendelenberg test	
	Measure leg length	
	Flexion	115°
	Extension	30°
	Abduction	50°
	Adduction	45°
	Internal rotation	45°
	External rotation	45°
Knee	Test for the presence of fluid	
	Test for instability: laterally (collateral ligaments) or anteroposteriorly (cruciate ligaments)	
	Flexion	135°
	Extension	10°
Ankle	Flexion (plantarflexion)	50°
	Extension (dorsiflexion)	20°
Foot	Inversion and eversion (subtalar joints)	
	Abduction and adduction (midtarsal joints)	
	Flexion at the metatarsophalangeal and interphalangeal joints	

Table 7.3 Examination of individual joints: lower limb

3. EXAMINATION OF OTHER SYSTEMS
Special attention must be paid to those systems frequently involved in rheumatic conditions.
  a. The skin: Table 7.4.

Localised rash	'Butterfly': SLE
	Periorbital: dermatomyositis
	Psoriasis: psoriatic arthropathy
	Keratoderma blenorrhagica: Reiter's disease
Generalised rash	Pink macular rash of Still's disease
	Erythema marginatum: rheumatic fever
	Drugs: gold, penicillamine
Ulcers	Leg: Felty's syndrome, rheumatoid disease
	Fingertips: progressive systemic sclerosis
	Rheumatoid disease, SLE, polyarteritis
Telangiectasia	Progressive systemic sclerosis, SLE
Nodules	See tex and page 96
Nails	Psoriasis, Reiter's disease
Hair	Alopecia: SLE (with or without cyclophosphamide)

Table 7.4 Skin signs associated with rheumatic disorders

  b. Mucous membranes:
    (i) Mouth ulcers: Reiter's disease (painless), systemic lupus erythematosus, Behçet's syndrome, Felty's syndrome, agranulocytosis (gold, phenylbutazone).
    (ii) Genital lesions (you would not be expected to examine for these in a short case): ulcers (Behçet's), circinate balanitis (Reiter's).
  c. Eyes: conjunctivitis (kerato-conjunctivitis sicca; acute Reiter's disease); episcleritis (rheumatoid disease); iritis (ankylosing spondylitis; Behçet's; recurrent Rei-

ter's; Still's disease); cataract (steroids); retinal cytoid bodies (systemic lupus erythematosus).
d. Splenomegaly and hepatomegaly: Still's disease; Felty's syndrome; systemic lupus erythematosus.

RHEUMATIC DISEASES

COMMON SHORT CASES

1. RHEUMATOID DISEASE

Sex incidence 3 females: 1 male. Age of onset: peak in the fifth decade.

Possible features

Joints
1. Acute symmetrical inflammatory polyarthropathy, classically affecting the metacarpophalangeal, proximal interphalangeal and lateral four metatarsophalangeal joints. Synovial hypertrophy and effusion result in typical spindle-shaped swelling of the fingers and swelling of the dorsum of the wrist. May also affect the distal interphalangeal joints, wrists, elbows, shoulders, upper cervical spine, temporo-mandibular joints, hips, knees, ankles, midtarsal joints, and crico-arytenoid joints (hoarseness, dysphagia).
2. Chronic disease (the usual presentation in a short case):
   a. Deformities:
      (i) Ulnar deviation at the metacarpophalangeal joints.
      (ii) 'Swan-neck' deformity: hyperextension at the proximal and fixed flexion deformity of the distal interphalangeal joint.
      (iii) Boutonnière deformity (button-hole): fixed flexion deformity of the proximal, with extension at the distal interphalangeal joint.
      (iv) Z-shaped adduction deformity of the thumb.
      (v) Flexion or valgus (rarely varus) deformities at the knee joints.
      (vi) Palmar subluxation of the metacarpophalangeal joints, or metatarsophalangeal (dorsal), or wrist joints (carpi lie anteriorly).
   b. Wasting of the small muscles of the hand.
   c. Rarely: rupture of the extensor tendons of the fingers, Baker's cyst formation and rupture.

Skin
1. Palmar erythema.
2. Subcutaneous nodules (25%): over pressure points, e.g. extensor surface of the elbows, achilles tendon, ischial tuberosities. May also occur in the hand, related to tendons.
3. Arteritis: nail-fold lesions; skin necrosis (e.g. leg ulcer); peripheral gangrene.

4. Maculopapular rash: e.g. gold, penicillamine treatment.
5. Thin atrophic skin: steroid therapy.

Nervous system
1. Spinal cord compression: due to subluxation of the cervical vertebrae, clasically at the atlanto-axial joints but may occur in the lower segments.
2. Cervical nerve root compression.
3. Entrapment neuropathy (e.g. carpal tunnel syndrome); mononeuritis multiplex (arteritis); symmetrical peripheral neuropathy (e.g. gold or chloroquine therapy).
4. Proximal myopathy (e.g. steroids), or myositis.

Eyes
1. Episcleritis.
2. Scleromalacia perforans.
3. Keratoconjunctivitis sicca.
4. Iatrogenic: cataract (steroids), retinal degeneration (chloroquine).

Respiratory system
1. Pleurisy; unilateral pleural effusion.
2. Diffuse interstitial fibrosis (may be clubbed).
3. Rheumatoid nodules (with coal-workers pneumoconiosus: Caplan's syndrome).

Cardiovascular system
1. Raynaud's phenomenon.
2. Cardiac involvement: pericarditis; constrictive pericarditis; aortic or mitral regurgitation; atrio-ventricular block (rheumatoid nodules)

Others
Anaemia; splenomegaly (15%; with neutropenia: Felty's syndrome); lymphadenopathy (10%; usually in areas draining inflamed joints); nephrotic syndrome (amyloidosis; gold or penicillamine therapy).

Complications
Septic arthritis; Baker's cyst rupture; osteoporosis; amyloidosis (3–5%).

2. ANKYLOSING SPONDYLITIS
Sex incidence 9 males : 1 female. Age of onset: peak in the third decade. 96% of cases have the HLA antigen B27.

Possible features

Joints
1. Advanced cases (the usual presentation in a short case): bony ankylosis of the whole spine results in severe thoracic kyphosis, with loss of lumbar lordosis and compensatory hyperextension of the neck ('poker back'; 'question-mark' posture). There is also limitation of chest expansion (costovertebral joints).

2. Early stages (rare short case):
   a. Diminution of movement of the lumbar spine (especially lateral flexion) and thoracic spine (rotation). Loss of the lumbar curve when standing erect; and failure to obliterate the lumbar lordosis on full flexion of the spine. Sacro-iliac irritability. (Identical features may be seen in psoriatic arthropathy, inflammatory bowel disease, and recurrent Reiter's disease).
   b. Asymmetrical peripheral arthritis (10–20%): usually involves the lower limb (e.g. hip, knee).
   c. Achilles tendinitis, plantar fasciitis.

Eyes   Sterile conjunctivitis; iritis (10–40%): commoner in those with peripheral joint involvement.

Others   Aortic regurgitation (1%); apical lung fibrosis (1%); inflammatory bowel disease (10%).

Complications   Amyloidosis; spinal cord compression (atlantoaxial subluxation; fracture of the rigid spine).

3. SYSTEMIC LUPUS ERYTHEMATOSUS

Sex incidence 9 females : 1 male. Age of onset: peak in the late teens, early 20's.

Possible features

Skin (the usual presentation in a short case)
1. Erythematous rash across the bridge of the nose and cheeks ('butterfly rash'); occasionally also on the upper trunk and arms (areas exposed to light). More common clinically are circumscribed, indurated red-purple plaques over the nose and cheeks, with scaling, telangiectases and follicular plugging.
2. Alopecia: scarring or non-scarring.
3. Raynaud's phenomenon.
4. Others: palmar erythema, or erythema around the finger-nails; maculopapular rash; purpura or ecchymoses; oral or leg ulceration; livedo reticularis; pigmentation; subcutaneous nodules; erythema multiforme.

Joints   Migratory polyarthralgia of the hands, wrists, knees or ankles. Aseptic necrosis of the hip. Rarely: deforming arthritis of the hands (due to tendon contractures).

Renal   Ranges from proteinuria to frank nephrotic syndrome, renal impairment to acute renal failure.

Nervous system   Psychosis; peripheral neuropathy; polymyositis; proximal myopathy (steroids).

Respiratory system	Pleurisy or pleural effusion; atelectasis; interstitial fibrosis.
Cardiovascular system	Pericarditis; cardiomyopathy; Libman-Sacks endocarditis (usually not diagnosed in life).
Others	Hepatic or splenic enlargement; generalised lymphadenopathy; cytoid bodies (soft exudates) in the retina, Sjögren's syndrome; anaemia, leucopenia, thrombocytopenia.
Drug-induced lupus	For example, hydrallazine, isoniazid, procainamide. Usually no renal or neurological involvement, and low titre of anti-DNA antibodies. Syndrome regresses after drug withdrawal.
Discoid lupus erythematosus	Chronic skin disease on the cheeks and bridge of the nose, with erythema, scaling, plugging of the sebaceous glands and scarring. There may also be marked alopecia. Only a small percentage progress to systemic disease.

4. PROGRESSIVE SYSTEMIC SCLEROSIS (SCLERODERMA)

Sex incidence 2 females : 1 male. Age of onset: 30–50 years.

Possible features

Skin (the usual presentation in a short case)	1. Hardened, thickened and immobile shiny skin, with oedema, loss of hair and pigmentation. Changes are usually maximal over the fingers (sclerodactyly; with or without atrophy (poikiloderma) or ulceration of the finger pulp), and the face (mask-like facies, and a pinched nose. Ask the patient to open her mouth: look for microstomia and fissures radiating from the mouth). There may be more extensive involvement of the arms and upper trunk ('suit of armour').
	2. Subcutaneous calcinosis: palpable nodules in the hands and extensor aspects of the elbows (if widespread: Thibierge-Wissenbach syndrome), which may ulcerate through the skin.
	3. Telangiectasia: usually accompany the skin changes on the hands, face and lips (and palate).
	4. Raynaud's phenomenon.
Joints	Inflammatory polyarthropathy affecting mainly the small joints of the hands. Together with the skin oedema give rise to the characteristic 'sausage fingers'.
Gastrointestinal system	Reduced motility of the oesophagus (peptic oesophagitis, dysphagia) and, less often, of the small intestine (diarrhoea, or steatorrhoea).

Respiratory system	Diffuse interstitial fibrosis (may lead to pulmonary hypertension or respiratory failure); overspill pneumonitis.
Cardiovascular system	Pericarditis or pericardial effusion; cardiac failure.
Renal failure	With or without hypertension.
Others	Sjögren's syndrome; myopathy; peripheral neuropathy.
Morphoea or linear scleroderma	Localised sclerodermatous lesion with a sharp line of demarcation from normal skin. Usually on the trunk or limbs. Does not progress to systemic sclerosis.
CREST syndrome	(calcinosis, Raynaud's phenomenon, oesophageal dysfunction, subcutaneous calcinosis and telangiectasia) More benign variant of progressive systemic sclerosis.

RARE SHORT CASES

1. GOUT

Possible features

1. Chronic gouty arthropathy (the usual presentation in a short case): features of osteoarthrosis in association with tophaceous swellings in and around affected joints. May also see tophi on the helix of the ear (very rarely also occur in the cornea, sclerae, renal pyramids and on heart valves).
2. Acute attack: tenderness and swelling, classically first affecting the metatarsophalangeal joint of the big toe (podagra). The overlying skin is warm, red and dry (wet in septic arthritis). Gout may attack any joint in the body, though only rarely the hips and shoulders.
3. Increased incidence of systemic hypertension, diabetes mellitus and ischaemic heart disease.

Causes

1. Primary: post-pubertal males and, less commonly, post-menopausal women.
2. Secondary:
   a. Reduced renal uric acid clearance: drugs (salicylates, thiazide diuretics, pyrazinamide); ketosis, glycogen storage diseases; alcohol excess; hyperparathyroidism, hypothyroidism; primary renal disease.
   b. Increased purine turnover: extensive psoriasis; myeloproliferative disorders (e.g. polycythaemia rubra vera, chronic myeloid leukaemia) and their treatment.
3. Acute attacks may be provoked by trauma, surgical operations, initiation of therapy (e.g. allopurinol), alcohol excess, or diuretic therapy.
4. Lesch-Nyhan syndrome: very rare X-linked recessive inborn error of metabolism (lack of the enzyme hypoxanthine guanine phosphoribosyltransferase).

Present in infancy with choreo-athetosis, spasticity, mental retardation and compulsive self-mutilation. Acute and chronic gouty arthropathy and tophi may occur.

2. PSORIATIC ARTHROPATHY

Equal sex incidence. Age of onset: 25–40 years. Affects 5% of cases of psoriasis.

Possible features

Joints   Four main patterns of involvement.
1. Asymmetrical involvement of the terminal interphalangeal joints of the fingers and toes, characteristically with psoriatic involvement of the overlying nails (commonest pattern).
2. Polyarthropathy indistinguishable from rheumatoid disease, though usually less extensive and more asymmetrical, and persistently seronegative.
3. Indistinguishable from ankylosing spondylitis.
4. Arthritis mutilans (main-en-lorgnette: opera glass hand): erosive destruction and resorption of the phalangeal heads results in telescoping of the soft tissues of the hands (very rare).

Skin and nail changes   Page 92. Rarely, the joint symptoms precede the psoriatic skin lesions by many years

3. REITER'S DISEASE

Almost exclusively affects males. Age of onset 20–30 years. 75% of cases have the HLA antigen B27.

Possible features   Develop following an attack of dysentery or non-specific diarrhoea, or non-specific urethritis.

Joints   1. Acute asymmetrical polyarthritis, usually affecting the lower limbs: knees, ankles, mid-tarsal, metatarsophalangeal and interphalangeal joints.
2. Achilles tendinitis or plantar fasciitis.
3. In recurrent attacks there is more prominent sacroiliitis and lumbar spine involvement, which are indistinguishable from classical ankylosing spondylitis.

Skin   Keratoderma blenorrhagica on the soles or palms (1%: may be difficult to distinguish from psoriasis); circinate balanitis; painless superficial mouth ulcers; nail involvement (subungual separation).

Eyes   Conjunctivitis (30%; with the acute attack) or iritis (with recurrent attacks).

Other features   Aortic incompetence; peripheral neuropathy, optic neuritis, meningo-encephalitis.

4. DEGENERATIVE JOINT DISEASE

a. Osteoarthrosis of peripheral joints
May be primary or secondary

Possible features
1. Bony (marginal osteophytes) rather than synovial swelling.
2. Pattern of involvement: that of the underlying cause in secondary osteoarthrosis. The most commonly affected joints in primary osteoarthrosis are:
   a. In the hand: distal and proximal interphalangeal joints (with or without Heberden's or Bouchard's nodes); metacarpophalangeal joints, and the first carpometacarpal joint ('square hand' appearance).
   b. Knee, hip and spine. Involvement of the wrist, elbow and shoulder is very rare in primary osteoarthrosis.

Causes
1. Primary or nodal multiple osteoarthrosis: autosomal dominant inheritance in females, recessive in males. Age of onset: 50 years and over. Clinical hallmark is involvement of the terminal interphalangeal joints, with Heberden's node formation.
2. Secondary
   — genetic factors: e.g. Marfan's syndrome, ochronosis, gout
   — endocrine abnormalities: e.g. acromegaly, hyperparathyroidism (chondrocalcinosis)
   — inflammatory arthropathies: e.g. rheumatoid disease, septic arthritis
   — anatomical abnormalities: e.g. congenital dislocation of the hip; avascular necrosis (e.g. sickle cell disease; steriod treatment); Paget's disease
   — neuropathic causes: e.g. Charcot's arthropathy: diabetes or leprosy (hands, feet), syringomyelia (upper limb), or neurosyphilis (lower limb)
   — trauma: e.g. pneumatic drill workers (elbows), heavy lifting (lumbar spine), athletes (knees)

b. Spondylosis and disc lesions (very rare short cases)

Possible features
1. Acute cervical disc protrusion:
   a. Neck held in a fixed position by muscle spasm; may be localised tenderness in the neck.
   b. May have neurological deficit (p. 29): due to root involvement (most commonly C5 or C6), or rarely to long tract involvement (posterior disc protrusion).

2. Cervical spondylosis:
   a. Limitation of neck movement.
   b. May have neurological deficit: most commonly C5 or C6.
3. Acute lumbar disc protrusion and lumbar spondylosis:
   a. Spine held in a position of scoliosis, tenderness over the affected area.
   b. Limited flexion of the spine.
   c. May have neurological deficit (p. 33): e.g. L5 or S1 root involvement.
   d. Painful limitation of straight leg raising (Lasègue's sign).

5. POLYARTERITIS NODOSA AND MICROSCOPIC POLYARTERITIS

The only features likely to be seen in a short case are mononeuritis multiplex or a vasculitic skin rash (e.g. livedo reticularis, skin necrosis, purpura).

Other features
1. Systemic disease: fever, polyarthritis.
2. Cardiovascular system: hypertension; palpable nodules on the arteries; coronary arteritis.
3. Gastrointestinal tract: mucosal ulceration, abdominal pain, intestinal infarction.
4. Kidney: haematuria, proteinuria, acute renal failure (necrotising glomerulitis).
5. Respiratory system: asthma; pulmonary cavitation, or haemorrhage.
6. Nervous system: cerebral infarction, encephalopathy.

6. JUVENILE CHRONIC ARTHRITIS (STILL'S DISEASE)

Only the long term sequelae of this disorder will be seen in a short case:

1. Growth retardation, either generalised (short stature) or local (e.g. receding chin: micrognathia).
2. Joint complications similar to adult rheumatoid disease.
3. Eye complications: irregular pupil due to adhesion of iris to anterior surface of the lens (previous uveitis), cataracts (steroids), band keratopathy.
4. Amyloidosis (3%): e.g. nephrotic syndrome.

Acute features   Three main patterns:
1. Systemic: high remittent temperature, evanescent maculopapular rash, generalised lymphadenopathy, hepatosplenomegaly, arthralgia (or no joint symptoms).
2. Polyarthritic: particularly the knees, wrists and carpi.
3. Pauci-articular (66% cases): risk of chronic iridocyclitis (10%).

7. SWOLLEN TENDER KNEE JOINT

Causes

Rheumatoid disease   May present with monarticular involvement.

Seronegative arthropathy

1. Ankylosing spondylitis: 10% of cases present with a peripheral arthropathy, usually in the lower limb.
2. Psoriatic arthropathy.
3. Reiter's disease.
4. Reactive arthritis: following a gastrointestinal infection with *Salmonella enteritis*, *Yersinia*, or *Campylobacter*.
5. Inflammatory bowel disease: Crohn's disease (20%), ulcerative colitis (12%). Acute monarthritis may occur with the onset of bowel disease, or during its course.
6. Whipple's disease: predominantly affects male patients. Arthritis or arthralgia occurs in 9% of cases, and may precede the bowel symptoms by many years. Other feature: lymphadenopathy.

Crystal arthropathy

1. Acute gout.
2. Acute pseudogout (pyrophosphate arthropathy; chondrocalcinosis); may be associated with hyperparathyroidism, haemochromatosis, acromegaly, Wilson's disease, diabetes mellitus, gout.

Infection

1. Septic arthritis: bacterial, tuberculous.
2. Gonorrhoea, meningococcal meningitis, bacterial endocarditis, acute rheumatic fever.
3. Viruses: rubella, hepatitis B.

Trauma   Epiphyseal fracture, haemarthrosis, foreign body, prepatellar bursitis (housemaids knee).

Very rare causes

Sarcoidosis   Erythema nodosum may be associated with arthritis of the ankles or knees.

Behçet's syndrome   Triad of recurrent oral and genital ulceration with iritis. Usually also have an arthritis or arthralgia, predominantly affecting large rather than small joints (e.g. knee). Other features: erythema nodosum, thrombophlebitis.

Relapsing polychondritis   Episodic inflammation of cartilaginous structures throughout the body (e.g. ears, joints, nose), together with inflammation of the eyes (conjunctivitis, iritis).

Multicentric reticulohistiocytosis Development of nodules in the skin and subcutaneous tissues (face, hands), resulting in facial disfigurement, and in the synovia and bones resulting in a destructive arthritis.

Pigmented villo-nodular synovitis Hypertrophied synovium with giant cells containing haemosiderin, and a bloody joint effusion.

Familial Mediterranean fever (relapsing polyserositis) Paroxysmal synovitis of the knees often a prominent feature. Restricted to people of Mediterranean ancestry, particularly Sephardic Jews and Armenians; usually have a family history. Onset in childhood or early adult life. Also have paroxysmal attacks of fever and abdominal pain (sterile peritonitis). Can lead to secondary amyloidosis.

8. 'THIS PATIENT HAS RAYNAUD'S PHENOMENON. EXAMINE HER'

The possibilities are:

1. Systemic connective tissue disorders: look for features of, e.g., rheumatoid disease, scleroderma, dermato- or polymyositis, SLE.
2. Atherosclerosis: e.g. subclavian or axillary artery (reduced brachial and radial pulses), or single digital arteries.
3. Buerger's disease: heavy smokers (men).
4. Thromboembolism: e.g. cervical rib syndrome (young women).
5. Physical injuries to the digital vessels: e.g. cold; vibrating tools.
6. Raynaud's disease: young women. Ulceration or gangrene never occur.
7. Miscellaneous: circulating cryoglobulins or cold agglutins; macroglobulinaemia; polycythaemia; vinyl chloride exposure.

8. Endocrine system

INTRODUCTION With the exception of diabetes mellitus, patients with endocrine or metabolic disorders are uncommon short cases. They are usually presented as a 'spot diagnosis' with the instruction 'Look at this patient's face' (e.g. Cushing's syndrome, acromegaly, hypothyroidism), or 'Examine the hands' (e.g. acromegaly), or 'Examine the neck' (e.g. goitre). Having made the diagnosis, you must be prepared with a list of the other features of that disorder.

ENDOCRINE AND METABOLIC DISORDERS

COMMON SHORT CASES

Possible features

1. DIABETES MELLITUS

Eyes Rubeosis of the iris (may cause glaucoma), cataract formation, diabetic retinopathy (p. 18).

Skin
1. Necrobiosis lipoidica diabeticorum (rare): reddish plaques with a central yellow area containing telangiectasia. May ulcerate, and then heal to leave a pale thin scar. Usually seen on the shins, and rarely on the arms and chest.
2. Insulin tumours or atrophy ('hollows') at the sites of repeated subcutaneous injections (upper arms, thighs).
3. Xanthoma diabeticorum (yellowish papules or nodules); moniliasis (mouth, balanitis); acute infections (e.g. boils); photosensitivity (chlorpropamide).
4. Leg ulcers (p. 136).

Arterial disease Peripheral vascular disease (absent pulses, trophic changes, gangrene: may require local amputation), and coronary artery disease.

Nervous system
1. Chronic peripheral sensory neuropathy: symmetrical, chiefly affecting the feet and legs. Loss of pain, vibration sensation, and deep tendon reflexes (e.g. ankle). May be complicated by diabetic foot (see below) and Charcot's arthropathy.
2. Subacute mixed neuropathy ('amyotrophy'): weakness and wasting, most often of the quadriceps muscle, with hyperaesthesia and some loss of pain

sensation over the front of the thigh; the ankle jerk is present, but the knee jerk absent.

3. Mononeuritis multiplex: e.g. foot drop, cranial nerve palsies (especially IIIn and VIn).

4. Autonomic neuropathy: impotence, diarrhoea, atonic bladder, postural hypotension, Argyll-Robertson pupils, gustatory sweating (facial sweating on eating certain foods: e.g. cheese).

Diabetic foot   For example, ulceration of the sole over pressure points. This occurs as a result of peripheral neuropathy and/or ischaemia, with or without added infection.

Kidneys   Glomerulosclerosis, pyelonephritis, renal papillary necrosis, chronic renal failure.

Causes

Commonest   Primary (idiopathic, essential) diabetes:
1. Insulin-dependent: may be associated with autoimmune disorders (e.g. Addison's disease, thyroid disease, pernicious anaemia, alopecia areata).
2. Non-insulin-dependent.

Rare   1. Secondary
   a. Endocrine: e.g. Cushing's syndrome, acromegaly, phaeochromocytoma, glucagonoma, hyperthyroidism.
   b. Pancreatic destruction: e.g. chronic pancreatitis, carcinoma, pancreatectomy, haemochromatosis ('bronze diabetes').
   c. Drugs: e.g. steroids, thiazide diuretics, oral contraceptives, diazoxide.
2. Associated with genetic syndromes: e.g. Friedreich's ataxia, dystrophia myotonica, Down's syndrome.

2. CUSHING'S SYNDROME

Possible features

General   Central fat hypertrophy (truncal obesity, buffalo hump, protruberant abdomen), with proximal limb wasting and weakness ('potato on matchsticks').

Face   Plethoric; 'moon face'; acne; hirsutism, with loss of scalp hair; pigmentation (with increased ACTH production).

Skin   Purple striae (especially on the abdominal wall); purpura (easy bruising); atrophic skin.

Chest   Kyphosis (osteoporotic vertebrae); hypertension.

Others | Diabetes mellitus, hypokalaemia, growth retardation in children; depression, psychoses, visual field defect (with a pituitary tumour); pathological fractures, aseptic necrosis of the hips.

Complications | Infection; coronary or cerebral artery disease; venous thrombosis.

Causes

Commonest | Corticosteroid or ACTH treatment: e.g. asthma, SLE, rheumatoid disease, renal transplantation.

Rare |
1. Pituitary-dependent bilateral adrenocortical hyperplasia (Cushing's disease). Basophil hyperplasia or adenoma of the pituitary gland. 10% of those patients who undergo bilateral adrenalectomy for Cushing's disease later develop excessive pigmentation (Nelson's syndrome).
2. Adrenal tumour: adenoma or carcinoma.
3. Ectopic ACTH production: e.g. oat cell bronchial carcinoma. Patients do not show the weight gain, typical moon face or pigmentation, but characteristically have a hypokalaemic alkalosis. With less aggressive ACTH-secreting tumours (e.g. thymomas, carcinoids), pigmentation is a prominent feature.

RARE SHORT CASES |
1. HYPERTHYROIDISM (THYROTOXICOSIS)
Sex incidence : 5 females : 1 male.

Possible features

Diffuse toxic goitre | Listen for a systolic bruit. Less commonly: toxic nodule, or toxic multinodular goitre.

Eyes | Exophthalmos (the sclera is visible above the lower eyelid; may be unilateral); lid retraction (the sclera is visible below the lower margin of the upper eyelid and the iris), and lid-lag. Rarely: external ophthalmoplegia (lateral or superior rectus muscles), periorbital oedema, conjunctivitis.

Skin |
1. Fine tremor of the outstretched fingers. Warm, moist palms.
2. Pretibial myxoedema (rare): areas of thickened ('orange-peel'), non-tender, bluish-red infiltration of the skin. Usually affects the shins or tops of the feet, but may also be seen on the hands. Only seen in Graves' disease; may still be present when the patient is euthyroid.

Nails	1. Onycholysis (10%).
	2. Thyroid acropachy: resembles clubbing, but there is no oedema of the nail-fold, and the thumb and index finger are the most severely affected. Only seen in Graves' disease.
Cardiovascular system	Sinus tachycardia, with a full volume pulse; atrial fibrillation.
Others	Proximal myopathy, brisk tendon reflexes, myaesthenia gravis, osteoporosis, psychoses; diarrhoea; gynaecomastia, diabetes mellitus; splenomegaly, lymphadenopathy (longstanding disease).

Causes

Common	— diffuse toxic goitre (Graves' disease): younger age group. Eye signs common. May be associated with other autoimmune diseases (e.g. vitiligo, pernicious anaemia, Addison's disease, diabetes mellitus, alopecia areata).
	— toxic nodular goitre (multinodular or uninodular): older age group. Eye signs rare. No association with autoimmune diseases.
Rare	— excess thyroid stimulating hormone (TSH) or TSH-like material: e.g. pituitary tumour, choriocarcinoma, hydatidiform mole.
	— exogenous administration of thyroxine: e.g. intentional self-administration, or overenthusiastic treatment of hypothyroidism.
	— transient: associated with thyroiditis (e.g. Hashimoto's, or subacute thyroiditis).

2. HYPOTHYROIDISM (MYXOEDEMA)

Possible features

Face	Typical facial appearance with pallor, periorbital puffiness, and loss of the lateral third of the eyebrows. May also see dry, brittle hair, with or without alopecia.
Goitre	May be present (see below).
Skin	Rough, dry and cold. Often has a slight yellow tinge (hyperlipidaemia). Onycholysis (rare), leuconychia.
Cardiovascular system	Sinus bradycardia. Rarely: cardiac failure, cardiomyopathy, pericardial effusion.
Nervous system	Dementia, cerebellar ataxia, deafness, peripheral neuropathy, entrapment neuropathy (e.g. carpal tunnel

syndrome), and delayed relaxation of the tendon reflexes.

Others   Weight gain; hoarse voice; arthritis (chondrocalcinosis); constipation (palpable sigmoid colon), ascites; anaemia; hypothermia (erythema ab igne on legs).

Features of associated organ-specific autoimmune diseases   For example, vitiligo, alopecia areata.

Causes

Common   — destruction of the thyroid gland: e.g. surgical removal (look for the scar), ^{131}I therapy
— autoimmune thyroiditis: following Hashimoto's disease (goitre), or spontaneous atrophy (no goitre). May be associated with other autoimmune diseases.

Rare   — reduced synthesis of thyroid hormones: e.g. iodine deficiency; goitrogenic drugs (e.g. carbimazole, lithium, phenylbutazone, iodides in cough medicine); dyshormonogenesis (with deafness: Pendred's syndrome)
— secondary to pituitary or hypothalamic disease
— agenesis: results in cretinism
— replacement of gland by carcinoma

3. GOITRE, OR 'LOOK AT THIS PATIENT'S THYROID GLAND'

Technique

Inspection   From the front, look at the patient's neck and ask him to swallow (if necessary, after giving him a sip of water). Look for a thyroidectomy scar (if present, suspect hypothyroidism, or hypoparathyroidism: Chvostek's sign, Trousseau's sign).

Palpation   1. Thyroid: stand behind the patient, and palpate with both hands. Alternatively, stand at his side and palpate with the index and middle fingers of one hand. Note the following:
a. Size: small (palpable, but not visible), medium (visible) or large (obvious, with an increase in the neck circumference).
b. Character: diffuse or nodular.
c. Tenderness: e.g. viral thyroiditis.
d. Mobility: especially any attachment to to the overlying skin, or to the sternomastoid muscles.
e. Retrosternal extension: feel in the suprasternal notch, and percuss over the upper sternum.
f. Tracheal deviation.

2. Palpate for enlarged cervical lymph glands: e.g. thyroid carcinoma, thyroiditis.

Auscultation If a diffuse nodular goitre is present, listen for a systolic bruit.

If indicated, briefly look for evidence of thyrotoxicosis or hypothyroidism

Causes

Common — simple non-toxic goitre: e.g. iodine deficiency, goitrogens (e.g. carbimazole, lithium, phenylbutazone), dyshormonogenesis (with deafness: Pendred's syndrome)
— diffuse toxic goitre (Graves' disease)
— autoimmune thyroiditis (Hashimoto's disease)

Rare — thyroid carcinoma: e.g. medullary carcinoma (may be associated with skin or mucous membrane neurinomas on the lip or eyelids, or in the mouth). Features which suggest a malignant goitre: asymmetry, hardness, hoarseness, fixation to the skin and underlying tissues
— other forms of thyroiditis: acute, subacute (de Quervain's), Riedel's (woody)
— infiltration: metastases, sarcoidosis, amyloidosis

4. ACROMEGALY
Excessive secretion of growth hormone from an eosinophil or chromophobe pituitary adenoma.

Possible features Overgrowth of soft tissues (skin, tongue, viscera) and bones.

Face Increase in size of the skull vault, supraorbital ridges and lower jaw (prognathism; teeth separation; reversed bite). Enlarged lips and tongue, broad nose, and exaggerated skin folds; the skin may be greasy and sweaty. Acne and hirsutism may also occur.

Limbs Broad spade-shaped hands and feet; carpal tunnel syndrome. Degenerative joint disease (knee, shoulder, hip joints). Chondrocalcinosis.

Chest Kyphosis (vertebral enlargement); gynaecomastia (with or without galactorrhoea); skin papillomata. Hypertension; cardiomyopathy.

Abdomen Hepatosplenomegaly, splenomegaly.

Nervous system	Visual field defects, optic atrophy; entrapment neuropathy (e.g. carpal tunnel syndrome).
Other endocrine or metabolic disorders	1. Diabetes mellitus (12%); abnormal glucose tolerance test (20%). 2. Diffuse or nodular goitre (22%). 3. Diabetes insipidus. 4. Hypopituitarism: hypogonadism. 5. Hypercalcaemia (12%), or hypercalcuria (20%): renal stones. May be part of the type I Multiple Endocrine Adenomatosis syndrome (MEA type I: with hyperparathyroidism, Zollinger-Ellison syndrome, and an adrenocortical tumour. MEA type II associates medullary carcinoma of the thyroid with phaeochromocytoma; primary hyperparathyroidism may also occur). 6. Type IV lipoproteinaemia.

5. ADRENOCORTICAL INSUFFICIENCY

Possible features

Hyperpigmentation	Due to adrenocorticotrophin (ACTH) excess, so only present in Addison's disease. Occurs in areas exposed to the sun, pressure areas (elbows, under straps or rings), buccal mucosa (gums, lips, inside cheeks), areolae of the nipples, skin creases (palms), and scars. May also have vitiligo.
Postural hypotension; tachycardia	
Others	Weight loss, tiredness, lethargy; loss of body hair in women.

Causes

Chronic	*1. Primary adrenocortical insufficiency (Addison's disease)* Common: autoimmune adrenalitis (may be associated with other autoimmune disorders) tuberculous destruction Rare: infarction or haemorrhage, metastases, sarcoidosis, amyloidosis, adrenalectomy. *2. Secondary adrenocortical insufficiency* Common: sudden withdrawal of steroids, or stress whilst on steroid therapy Rare: pituitary or hypothalamic disease (p. 123).
Acute	e.g. Waterhouse Friedrichsen syndrome (meningococcal septicaemia).

6. HYPOPITUITARISM

Possible features Determined by the pattern of hormone deficiency present (whether single or multiple), the stage in growth and development when the hypopituitarism develops, and any associated pressure symptoms (if due to a tumour).

Gonadotrophins 1. Children: failure to enter puberty; eunuchoid skeletal proportions.
2. Adults: impotence, infertility; progressive loss of secondary sexual characteristics (e.g. stop shaving; atrophy of breasts and genitalia); skin changes (fine wrinkles at the corners of the mouth and eyes).

Growth hormone 1. Children: short stature.
2. Adults: fasting hypoglycaemia.

Thyrotrophin Features of hypothyroidism, though less dramatic; e.g. no coarsening of the facies.

Adrenocorticotrophin (no effect on aldosterone secretion) Pale smooth ('babylike') skin, and pale areolae of the nipples; fasting hypoglycaemia.

Pressure effects Bitemporal hemianopia, optic atrophy.

Causes — tumours: pituitary (primary or secondary); supra-sellar (e.g. craniopharyngioma; meningioma)
— granulomas: e.g. sarcoidosis
— infarction: e.g. post-partum (Sheehan's syndrome)
— iatrogenic: e.g. irradiation, hypophysectomy
— very rare developmental abnormalities: e.g. Kallman's syndrome (with anosmia, and occasionally colour blindness and nerve deafness)

Diabetes insipidus Polyuria, polydipsia

Causes 1. Cranial: primary (hereditary or idiopathic forms), or secondary (head injury; causes of hypopituitarism).
2. Nephrogenic: primary (hereditary), or secondary (e.g. hypercalcaemia, hypokalaemia, lithium treatment).

7. PORPHYRIA

Hepatic

Acute intermittent porphyria Autosomal dominant inheritance. Acute attacks, usually followed by complete remission. Attacks precipitated by drugs (e.g. barbiturates, contraceptive pill), alcohol, hormonal factors (e.g. pregnancy), acute infections, and dieting.

Features   Abdominal pain, vomiting, constipation; peripheral neuropathy (e.g. wrist or foot drop: 60%); sinus tachycardia, hypertension (70%); psychoses. Urine darkens on standing (oxidation of excess porphobilinogen). No skin involvement.

Cutaneous hepatic porphyria (porphyria cutanea tarda; 'symptomatic porphyria')   Non-acute. Usually secondary to alcoholic liver disease.

Features   Photosensitive skin eruptions (erythema, vesicles, bullae), which heal with scarring (face, neck, forearms, hands). Hyperpigmentation, hirsutism and increased fragility of the skin (positive Nikolsky's sign). Excess uroporphyrin in the urine.

Erythropoietic   Very rare; e.g. erythropoietic protoporphyria, congenital porphyria.

Features   Severe photosensitive skin lesions, with gross scarring and disfigurement; red-staining of the teeth, and hirsutism ('werewolf'). Excess urinary uroporphyrin 1 and coproporphyrin 1.

8. TALL STATURE

Causes

Marfan's syndrome   Autosomal dominant inheritance.

Features   1. Musculo-skeletal: overgrowth of the long bones results in disproportionately long limbs (arm span is greater than the height). High, full forehead; narrow, high-arched palate. 'Pigeon-breast' chest, with kyphoscoliosis. Long ('spider') fingers (arachnodactyly) and toes; when the thumb is enclosed in a closed fist it protrudes beyond the medial border of the hand (Steinberg's sign).
2. Ocular: upwards lens dislocation, iridodonesis ('wobbly' iris: also seen following cataract removal).
3. Cardiovascular: aortic regurgitation, mitral valve prolapse syndrome, atrial septal defect; aortic aneurysm formation, or dissection.
4. Excessive joint laxity ('double-jointed'); hypotonia.

Homocystinuria   Autosomal recessive inheritance. Inborn error of methionine metabolism.

Features   1. Physical appearance similar to Marfan's syndrome. May also have lens dislocation (usually downward).
2. Recurrent thromboses.
3. Mentally handicapped.

Klinefelter's syndrome: XXY

Features 1. Eunuchoid proportions; gynaecomastia. Varying degrees of hypogonadism (reduced facial hair; female distribution of body hair). Small soft testicles.
2. May be mentally subnormal.

Gigantism; hyperthyroidism; familial tall stature

9. SHORT STATURE

Causes

Turner's syndrome (gonadal dysgenesis): XO

Features 1. Short, stocky build. Webbing of the neck (40%). Shield-shaped chest, with small, widely-spaced nipples. Cubitus valgus (increased carrying angle). Sexually immature (infantile external genitalia). Pigmented naevi.
2. Face: epicanthic folds; micrognathia; deformed or low-set ears; low posterior hair line.
3. Hands: swelling of the dorsum; short fourth meta-carpal bone.
4. Others: may be associated with coarctation of the aorta, horseshoe kidneys.

Achondroplasia Autosomal dominant. Short limbs (more marked proximally than distally: humerus and femur) with relatively normal sized spine (often kyphotic). Large head, with prominent forehead and depressed nasal bridge. Normal sexual deve(ment and intelligence.

Osteogenesis imperfecta Autosomal dominant. Bowing of the legs, pectus excavatum, kyphoscoliosis; hyperextensible joints. Other features: blue sclerae, otosclerosis.

Endocrine Associated with precocious puberty (due to early epiphyseal closure); Cushing's syndrome; growth hormone deficiency; hypothyroidism.

Systemic disease Malabsorption, renal or hepatic disease, hypoxaemia (e.g. cyanotic congenital heart disease).

Starvation; emotional deprivation

Familial short stature Growth delay.

Other syndromes e.g. mucopolysaccharidoses.

10. HYPOTHERMIA

Core temperature below 35°C. The patient is usually presented in a space blanket.

Features
1. Progressive impairment of consciousness.
2. Cardiovascular: bradycardia, hypotension, increased myocardial irritability (atrial fibrillation), J-wave on ECG.
3. Respiratory: reduced cough reflex, cold-induced bronchorrhoea.
4. Others: polyuria (risk of hypovolaemia), pancreatitis (usually only biochemical), hypoglycaemia, acidosis; shift of oxyhaemoglobin dissociation curve to the left (increased affinity for oxygen).

Causes
— accidental: elderly, alcoholics, epileptics
— endocrine: hypothyroidism, hypopituitarism
— damage to the heat-conserving mechanisms in the posterior hypothalamus: e.g. neoplasm, trauma, embolism
— drugs: e.g. sedatives, chlorpromazine
— skin disorders: e.g. erythroderma, burns

9. Face and neck

EXAMINATION OF THE FACE Patients with abnormal facial signs are common short cases. They are often 'spot diagnoses', which lead on to a search for, or discussion of, other features of that condition. Many of the features and disorders listed below have already been mentioned in previous chapters (cross-references are given).

'EXAMINE THIS MAN'S FACE' This should include the following:

1. GENERAL: IS THE DIAGNOSIS OBVIOUS?
For example:

Congenital disorder

Down's syndrome Usually trisomy of chromosome 21.

Features
1. Craniofacial: brachycephaly, flat-face, low-set ears. The eyes have a laterally directed upward slope; epicanthic folds; Brushfield spots (greyish white areas of depigmentation at the periphery of the iris). Macroglossia; 'scrotal tongue'.
2. Skeletal:
   a. Short stature.
   b. Hands: broad flat hands; shortening and incurving of the little finger (clinodactyly). Characteristic dermatoglyphic patterns: single palmar crease, distal axial tri-radius, and ulnar loops on the fingers.
   c. Feet: wide space between the first and second toes.
3. Nervous system: muscle hypotonia; hypermobile joints; deafness; mental subnormality.
4. Cardiovascular: ventricular or atrial septal defect.
5. Others: developmental gastrointestinal defects (e.g. duodenal atresia, imperforate anus); male infertility; infections; leukaemia.

Dystrophia myotonica (p. 46)

Endocrine disorder Cushing's syndrome (p. 117); acromegaly (p. 121); myxoedema (p. 119), thyrotoxicosis (p. 118).

Neurological disorder Cerebrovascular accident; Parkinson's disease (p. 42); facial palsy (p. 14); involuntary movements (e.g. phenothiazines; p. 37).

Collagen disease	Systemic lupus erythematosus (p. 108); progressive systemic sclerosis (p. 109).
Skin disease	Acne vulgaris (p. 94), rosacea (p. 94): squamous-cell or basal-cell (rodent ulcer) carcinoma, herpes zoster of Va.
Skeletal disease	For example:
Paget's disease of bone	Large head with frontal bossing (also seen in rickets, and congenital syphilis). May be complicated by cranial nerve lesions (e.g. optic atrophy, deafness), or spinal cord compression (basilar invagination). Other complications: fractures, heart failure, sarcomatous change.
Previous Still's disease	Receding chin (micrognathia: p. 113).
Renal disorder	For example, partial lipodystrophy: symmetrical loss of subcutaneous fat from the face and arms. Associated with mesangiocapillary nephritis (dense deposit type), and the nephritic factor.

2. LOOK AT THE HAIR FOR:
a. Colour: e.g. white in pernicious anaemia.
b. Alopecia: page 101.

3. EXAMINE THE EYES AND EYELIDS:
page 16.

4. LOOK AT THE NOSE FOR:

Size	Enlarged in acromegaly, sarcoidosis (lupus pernio: p. 79), rosacea (rhinophyma: p. 94).
Shape	For example: collapsed bridge ('saddle-nose')
Causes (all rare)	— polychondritis (p. 114) — polyarteritis (p. 113) — congenital syphilis. Other features: frontal bossing ('hot cross bun' skull), failure of development of the maxilla ('bulldog facies'), interstitial keratitis, Hutchinson's teeth, Moon's molars, rhagades, deafness, and sabre tibia. — others: trauma; achondroplasia (p. 125).
Nodules	For example, adenoma sebaceum (tuberose sclerosis: p. 97).

5. LOOK AT THE CHEEKS FOR:

Facial erythema with a rash

Common causes
— systemic lupus ertyhematosus (p. 108)
— progressive systemic sclerosis (p. 109)
— Cushing's syndrome with acne (p. 117)

Rare causes
— rosacea (p. 94)
— light sensitivity (p. 95): porphyria, drugs
— erysipelas

**Facial erythema or plethora
without a rash**

Common causes
— malar flush (mitral stenosis)
— polycythaemia (e.g. polycythaemia rubra vera; chronic bronchitis)

Rare causes
— carcinoid syndrome: initially paroxysmal erythema, later fixed. Other features: page 66
— superior vena caval obstruction (p. 79)

**Spider naevi (p. 81),
telangiectasia (p. 81), hirsutism
(p. 102)**

Pigmentation (p. 198)

6. LOOK AT THE LIPS FOR:

Angular cheilitis   Dentures, iron-deficiency anaemia.

Peri-oral freckle-like melanotic pigmentation   Peutz-Jegher syndrome (p. 98).

Infections (very rare short cases)   For example, recurrent herpes simplex, impetigo.

7. LOOK AT THE TONGUE FOR:

Enlargement   Acromegaly (p. 121), amyloidosis, Down's syndrome (p. 127).

Wasting, fasciculation, or weakness (p. 98)

Colour change   For example, 'raw beef' in B12 deficiency (p. 45)

Telangiectasia   May also be present on the lips, buccal mucosa, palate and under the tongue (common short case).

Common causes   — progressive systemic sclerosis (p. 109)

— hereditary haemorrhagic telangiectasia (Osler-Rendu-Weber disease): autosomal dominant inheritance. Other features: bleeding from telangiectasia in the gastrointestinal tract or from pulmonary arteriovenous fistulae; splenomegaly.

Rare causes — discoid lupus erythematosus (p. 109)

Changes in its character For example, atrophic papillae (iron deficiency anaemia), scrotal tongue (Down's syndrome: p. 127), geographical tongue, black hairy tongue (antibiotics).

Ulcers See below.

8. LOOK AT THE GUMS, BUCCAL MUCOSA AND PALATE FOR:

Gum hyperplasia

Common causes — pregnancy
— drugs: phenytoin, contraceptive pill

Rare causes — scurvy
— leukaemia
— heavy metals: mercury

Pigmentation

Common cause — normal racial pigmentation

Rare causes — Addison's disease (p. 122)
— heavy metals: mercury, bismuth, or lead (blue line); arsenic, silver
— antimalarials: chloroquine, mepacrine

Ulcers (very rare short case)

Causes — oral carcinoma
— infections: bacterial (e.g. Vincent's organism, syphilis), viral (e.g. herpes simplex, zoster), or fungal (e.g. candidiasis)
— haematological: iron, B12 or folate deficiency; agranulocytosis (leukaemia; phenylbutazone, gold); Felty's syndrome (p. 107)
— skin diseases: pemphigus vulgaris (p. 96), dermatitis herpetiformis (p. 96), erythema multiforme (Stevens-Johnson syndrome: p. 95), lichen planus (p. 93)
— collagen disease: Reiter's disease (p. 111), systemic

lupus erythematosus (p. 108), Behçet's syndrome (p. 114)
— others: vasculitis (e.g. Wegener's granulomatosis); Crohn's disease; idiopathic (aphthous)

White patches

Causes   1. Lichen planus (p. 93).
2. Leukoplakia.
3. Candidiasis: may be removed by scraping. May be associated with:
   — changes in oral flora: antibiotics, steroids
   — dentures
   — xerostomia: Sjögren's syndrome, anti-Parkinsonian drugs
   — T-cell deficiency: leukaemia, immunosupressive drugs
   — iron deficiency anaemia
   — diabetes mellitus, hypoparathyroidism, Addison's disease, pregnancy.

High-arched palate   Marfan's syndrome (p. 124).

Nodules, tumours (very rare short cases)   9. LOOK AT THE TEETH FOR (very rare short cases):

Colour   Yellow-brown (smoking, tetracyclines, iron), or red discolouration (congenital erythropoietic porphyria).

Shape   Hutchinson's incisors (barrel-shaped, with notched incisal edges), Moon's molars (hypoplastic): features of congenital syphilis (look for rhagades: radiating scars on the lips. Other features: p. 128).

10. LOOK FOR PAROTID SWELLING

Common causes   — alcoholic cirrhosis (p. 85).
— Sjögren's syndrome (xerostomia with extensive dental caries; may be associated with rheumatoid disease or SLE).

Rare causes   — mumps
— drugs: methyldopa, guanethidine, clonidine
— sarcoid (with uveitis, facial palsy and fever: Heerfordt's syndrome: p. 79)
— lymphoma, leukaemia (Mikulicz's syndrome)
— parotid tumour or abscess; tuberculosis

11. LOOK AT THE EARS FOR:

Tophi (p. 110)

Vesicles on the pinna   Herpes zoster involving the facial nerve (Ramsey-Hunt syndrome). Other features: unilateral VIIn palsy, ulcers on the palate.

Slate blue pigmentation of the cartilage (and wax)   Ochronosis (alkaptonuria): autosomal recessive inheritance. Lack of the liver enzyme homogentisic acid oxidase. Urine darkens on standing.

NB: You are not likely to be asked to use an auriscope in a short case.

'EXAMINE THIS PATIENT'S NECK'   Rare short case

Technique   Examine for the following:

Thyroid gland   Page 120.

Cervical lymphadenopathy   Stand behind the patient and palpate with both hands. Remember to feel for both the occipital and supra-clavicular groups of nodes.

Causes
1. Regional lymphadenopathy: local infection (look in the mouth for oral sepsis; tuberculosis), neoplasm (e.g. thyroid, nasopharynx).
2. Generalised lymphadenopathy:
   — lymphoma, chronic lymphatic leukaemia
   — infection: bacterial (e.g. tuberculosis, secondary syphilis), viral (e.g. infectious mononucleosus), parasitic (toxoplasmosis)
   — collagen disease: rheumatoid disease (p. 106), juvenile chronic arthritis (p. 113), SLE (p. 108)
   — metastases
   — sarcoidosis (p. 79), drug reaction (e.g. phenytoin)

Jugular venous pressure   Page 50.

Carotid artery   Pulse rate, rhythm and volume. Listen for any bruits.

10. Arms

EXAMINATION OF THE ARMS AND HANDS

Patients with signs in the arms or hands are very common short cases. The abnormalities seen are usually in the nervous system (e.g. peripheral neuropathy (p. 40), carpal tunnel syndrome (p. 40), Parkinson's disease (p. 42)), or in the joints (e.g. rheumatoid disease: p. 106), and lead on to a search for other features of that disorder, or a discussion of other causes of a particular sign. There are also a number of very rare but benign conditions which are often used (e.g. dystrophia myotonica (p. 46), benign essential tremor (p. 36), syringomyelia (p. 44)). Although directed to the upper limb by the examiner, remember to look at the face for possible clues (e.g. Parkinsonian facies, thyrotoxic eye signs, acromegalic facies, Down's syndrome).

TECHNIQUE

This should include the following:

Inspection

Look for:
1. Joint swelling or deformity, and note its distribution: e.g. rheumatoid disease (p. 106), nodal osteoarthrosis (Heberden's nodes: p. 112), psoriatic arthropathy (involvement of the terminal interphalangeal joints and finger-nails: p. 111).
2. Muscle wasting: e.g. intrinsic hand muscles (p. 28), outer half of the thenar eminence (p. 27), deltoids (facio-scapulo-humeral dystrophy: (p. 46).
3. Abnormal posture: e.g. 'claw hand' (pp. 27 and 29), 'porter's tip' position (p. 29), Dupuytren's contracture (pp. 81 and 86).
4. Involuntary movements (p. 35): e.g. Parkinson's disease.
5. Skin changes (p. 91): e.g. spider naevi (p. 81), subcutaneous nodules (p. 96); violaceous rash over the dorsum of the fingers (dermatomyositis: p. 41); tight, shiny skin (progressive systemic sclerosis: p. 109); increased (p. 98) or decreased pigmentation (p. 97).
6. Nail changes (p. 100): e.g. clubbing; nail-fold or splinter haemorrhages (trauma, rheumatoid disease (p. 106), bacterial endocarditis (p. 67), dermatomyositis (p. 41), polyarteritis (p. 113)).

7. Swelling: e.g. lymphoedema (previous mastectomy, neoplastic involvement of the axillary nodes. Chronic forms may be complicated by sarcomatous change of the skin).

8. Abnormal shape: e.g. spade-like (acromegaly: p. 121), clinodactyly (Down's syndrome: p. 127), arachnodactyly (Marfan's syndrome: p. 124).

Palpation

1. Examine the peripheral pulses: page 49.
2. Examine the arms neurologically: page 24.
3. Feel for axillary lymphadenopathy.
4. Examine the joints (if indicated): page 104.

11. Legs

EXAMINATION OF THE LEGS

Less commonly asked than examination of the arms. The most likely abnormalities seen are either neurological (e.g. multiple sclerosis (p. 43), peripheral neuropathy (p. 40)), or vascular (e.g. diabetes mellitus (p. 116), leg ulcers)).

'EXAMINE THIS PATIENT'S LEGS'

This should include the following:

Inspection

Look for:

Joint swelling or deformity

For example, swollen knee joint (p. 114), Charcot's arthropathy (p. 112), pes cavus (Friedreich's ataxia (p. 44), peroneal muscular atrophy (p. 45)).

Bone deformity

For example, leg shortening (polio), bowing of the tibia ('sabre tibia') or femur (Paget's disease of bone, syphilis), loss of toes (previous amputation; e.g. peripheral vascular disease).

Enlargement of the calves

Common cause
— deep venous thrombosis

Rare causes
— ruptured popliteal (Baker's) cyst
— Duchenne muscular dystrophy (p. 47).

Swelling of the ankles

Common cause
— oedema (e.g. heart failure, anaemia, hypoproteinaemia)

Rare causes
— lymphoedema (hereditary: e.g. Milroy's disease; malignant nodes in both groins; filariasis)
— myxoedema (p. 119)

Muscle wasting

For example, of the quadriceps (proximal myopathy: p. 41), or calves (peroneal muscular atrophy: p. 45).

Abnormal posture

For example, foot drop (p. 34), joint contracture.

Skin changes (p. 91)   For example:

1. Leg ulcers (common short case)

Common causes
- venous: post-thrombotic, or primary venous incompetence. Gently shelving edge with a flat base, usually over the medial or occasionally the lateral malleolus. Other features: surrounding purpura, pigmentation, eczema, oedema, and liposclerosis (resultant fibrosis and scarring produces an 'inverted champagne bottle' appearance). May be complicated by malignancy (Marjolin's ulcer).
- ischaemia: atheroma (with or without hypertension, diabetes mellitus). Painful, 'punched-out' ulcer with steeply shelving edges, usually above the malleolus, or on the dorsum or sole of the foot. Other features: trophic changes (shiny skin, with loss of hair; cyanosed or necrotic toes); check for absent peripheral pulses (may be present in diabetes).
- neuropathy (trophic ulcers): diabetes mellitus. Painless, 'punched-out' ulcers, usually on the soles. Other features: loss of pain sensation, joint deformity (Charcot's arthropathy).

Rare causes
- ischaemia: Buerger's disease; vasculitis (rheumatoid disease, Felty's syndrome, polyarteritis); thrombosis or embolism; blood dyscrasias (hyperviscosity syndromes, cryoglobulinaemia, sickle cell disease, hereditary spherocytosis, polycythaemia, paroxysmal nocturnal haemoglobinuria)
- malignancy: squamous cell carcinoma (e.g. Marjolin's ulcer)
- neuropathy: spina bifida, tabes dorsalis (p. 46), leprosy
- infections: gumma, tuberculosis (erythema induratum), leishmaniais
- necrobiosis lipoidica diabeticorum (p. 116)
- pyoderma gangrenosum: inflammatory bowel disease, benign monoclonal gammopathy, rheumatoid disease, leukaemia. Large ulcer with bluish, undermined and irregular edge and central necrosis. May also occur on the face, trunk or upper limbs.
- hypertensive (Marterell's ulcer): painful, superficial ulceration of red-blue purpuric plaques, usually on the antero-lateral aspect of the leg below the knee

2. Trophic changes: shiny skin, with loss of hair; cyanosed or necrotic toes.
3. Rash: e.g. livedo reticularis (p. 113), erythema ab igne.
4. Hyperkeratosis of the feet (may affect the hands)

Common cause
- psoriasis

Rare causes — keratoderma blenorrhagica
— chronic arsenic ingestion (old treatment for syphilis)
— vitamin A deficiency
— tylosis (association with tendency to develop oesophageal carcinoma)

Palpation 1. Examine the peripheral pulses: page 49.
2. Examine the legs neurologically: page 30.
3. If indicated, examine particular joints: page 105.

Bibliography

GENERAL   Mason M, Swash M (eds) 1980 Hutchinson's clinical methods, 17th edn. Balliere Tindall and Cassell, London

Boucheir I A D, Morris J S (eds) 1982 Clinical skills, 2nd edn. WB Saunders, London

Zatouroff M 1976 A colour atlas of physical signs in general medicine. Wolfe, London

Beck E R, Francis J L, Souhami R L 1982 Tutorials in differential diagnosis, 2nd edn. Pitman Medical, London

Burton J L 1978 Aids to postgraduate medicine, 3rd edn. Churchill Livingstone, Edinburgh

Parfrey P S, Cunningham J 1980 Slide interpretation in postgraduate medicine. Oxford University Press, Oxford

NERVOUS SYSTEM   Patten J 1977 Neurological differential diagnosis. Harold Starke, London

Parsons M 1983 A colour atlas of clinical neurology. Wolfe, London

Glasspool M 1982 Atlas of ophthalmology. MTP, Lancaster

CARDIOVASCULAR SYSTEM   Turner R W D 1972 Auscultation of the heart. Churchill Livingstone, Edinburgh

RESPIRATORY SYSTEM   James D G, Studdy P R 1981 A colour atlas of respiratory diseases. Wolfe, London

ABDOMEN   Sherlock S, Summerfield J A 1979 A colour atlas of liver diseases. Wolfe, London

SKIN   Sneddon L B, Church R E 1976 Practical dermatology, 3rd edn. Arnold, London

Fry L 1978 Dermatology, an illustrated guide, 2nd edn. Update books, London

JOINTS   Currey H L F (ed) 1980 Mason and Currey's clinical rheumatology, 3rd edn. Pitman Medical, London

ENDOCRINE SYSTEM   Hall R, Evered D, Green R 1979 A colour atlas of endocrinology. Wolfe, London

Oakley W G, Pyke D A, Taylor K W 1978 Diabetes

and its management. Blackwell Scientific Publi-
cations, Oxford

RADIOLOGY   Hind C R K 1983 X-ray interpretation for MRCP.
Pitman Medical, London

Index